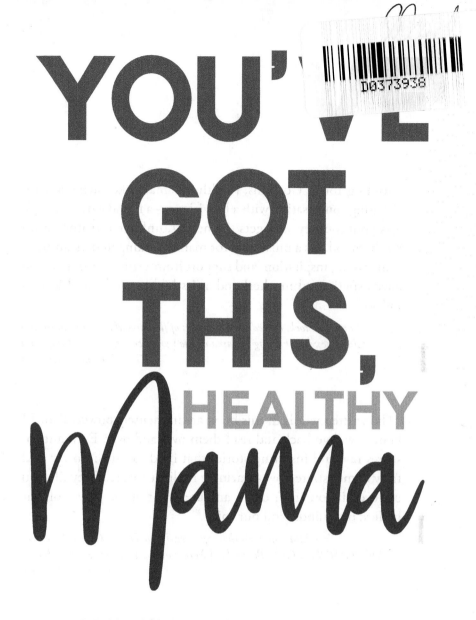

YOU'VE GOT THIS, *Mama* HEALTHY

A MOTHER'S GUIDE TO EMBRACING CHANGE
AND LIVING A HOLISTIC LIFE

"Reading You've Got This, Healthy Mama is like having a soul-cleansing conversation with a best friend—a friend who gets you, gets your journey, and gets the honest, unfiltered truths about motherhood. It's a must-read for mamas seeking understanding, compassion, inspiration, and support from a tribe of women who have experienced motherhood at its highest peaks and lowest valleys."

~ Christine Stock, copyeditor for writers of fiction and creative nonfiction
Christine Stock Editing | Mama of one | www.christinestockediting.com
IG: @christinestockediting

"The written words in this book are immensely powerful and I know I will go back and read them over and over. Each author shares raw and inspiring stories that hold so much power and truly demonstrate how amazingly resilient we are. They lift you up, even if you aren't down and are proof of the power of our bodies, our minds, and our spirit."

~ Kim Vopni, Author, Speaker, Pelvic Health Coach, President
Pelvienne Wellness Inc & Bellies Inc | Mama of two | www.vaginacoach.com
IG: @vaginacoach

"Finally, a book that truly touches on the lived experiences of women and MOMS. A collection of truth, healing and overcoming obstacles with fierce determination and perseverance. A must-read for every MOM and MOM-to-be."

~ Sandra Zichermann, Ph.D., Founder of The MOM Rant
Professor | MC/Host | Parenting Expert | MOM of three | momrant.com
IG: @TheMOMRant

"Each story resonated with me because I could see myself in them. The book left me inspired, motivated and ready to take on my own health goals as a busy mama of two!"

~ Sandra Everets, BScN, Registered Nurse
Owner of The Mama Coach—Halton Region| Mama of two
IG @sandrathemamacoach

"I am grateful to the strong and brave mamas who shared their personal motherhood journeys in You've Got This Mama. After reading each and every story I felt stronger, worthy and less alone. It reminded me to show myself more love, kindness, and compassion. To nourish my mind, body, and spirit. To know that I'm not alone with my feelings or emotions and that I'm a good mama. Thank you from the bottom of my heart for this gift, I will highly recommend it to every mama I know."

~ Jenny Kalynuik, Blogger
Creator of Little Lunch Love | Mama of two | IG @littlelunchlove

"Part of our human condition is to feel like what we're feeling, we're feeling in isolation. The essays in You've Got This, Healthy Mama shine a powerful light on the fact that we are all having a shared experience; that light allows the reader to become aware that they are never alone, find the comfort and community they seek, and begin to move on with the knowledge that they are a bigger part of a much bigger whole than they knew possible."

Leisse Wilcox, Professional Human + Real Life Adult
Speaker | Coach | Mom of three | IG: leissewilcox
Writer, and creator of To Call Myself Beloved: the Podcast with Leisse Wilcox

YOU'VE GOT THIS, HEALTHY Mama

A MOTHER'S GUIDE TO EMBRACING CHANGE AND LIVING A HOLISTIC LIFE

SABRINA GREER *featuring The Mama Tribe*

DAPHNE KOSTOVA · JENNIFER KALEY SMITS · STEPHANIE MOODY
NAOMI HAUPT · MELISSA SMITH · TARA BUTTERWICK
HILLARY DINNING · AMANDA ARCHIBALD · TANIA JANE MORAES-VAZ
MONA SHARMA · ANDREA TAYLOR · CHRISTINA WHELAN CHABOT
JODI DECLE · DANIELLE WILLIAMS · JUSTINE DOWD
MARIA BLACKLEY · SHAYROZ KHOSLA · LEISHA LAIRD

Published & Printed in Canada, for Global Distribution by YGTMama Media Co.

www.ygtmamamedia.co

For more information email: sabrina@ygtmama.com

ISBN trade paperback: 978-1-9990188-2-5

ebook: 978-1-9990188-7-0

To order additional copies of this book: sabrina@ygtmama.com

Table of Contents

SEVENTEEN 269

My Journey in the Raw
Shayroz Khosla

EIGHTEEN 283

Where Magic Dwells
Leisha Laird

FINAL THOUGHTS 293

Sabrina Greer

AUTHOR BIOS

Our children and those who matter will see our battle scars as beauty marks.

~ Sabrina Greer
@ygtmama

Introduction

Sabrina Greer

Health. *What is health?* The World Health Organization defines **health** as a "state of complete physical, mental, and social well-being, and not merely the absence of disease or infirmity." This definition made sense to me but still seemed rather vague. We hear the term "healthy" and see the concept of "health" *everywhere* we go. The wellness industry is currently a 4.2 trillion dollar industry and is spreading like wildfire.[1] There seems to be no age restriction on wanting to be *healthy*—it doesn't matter where you're from or what you do, health is becoming a top priority across the board.

What are the real answers when it comes to optimal health, though? *Is it meatless Mondays? Veganism? The Ketogenic diet? Paleo? Atkin's? Raw Food? No butter? More butter? Butter in my coffee? Coffee is good for my heart, right? Or is it red wine? Wait, **no** alcohol is obviously healthier? How many Weight Watchers points is that? Is that suited to my blood type? My menstrual cycle? Intermittent fasting? Did I hear something about a cookie diet? Will training for triathlons make me healthy? High Intensity Interval Training (HIIT)? Spin classes? Cardio? Low-impact walking? Doctor Ho's* *electrotherapy machine? Do I need to get a stripper pole? Or is it no genetically modified organisms (GMOs) in my food and products? What are GMOs? Strictly organic food? A magic pill or supplement? Lemon water with cayenne pepper and maple syrup?* It is seriously panic attack inducing. The amount of accessible information pertaining to health and wellness is plentiful, highly contradictory, and completely overwhelming. I found another definition for **health** from the Merriam-Webster dictionary that resonated: *Health is the condition of being **sound** in **body**, **mind**, and **spirit**.* This definition felt good to me, like something I could get on board with. Because being *sound* essentially means being capable. *Capable* of movement. *Capable* of making good decisions. *Capable* of common sense. *Capable* of listening to our body's signals.

As someone who worked as a fashion model for nearly two decades, my perception of *health* was always a tad skewed. I remember traveling to Taiwan on my first modeling contract when I was sixteen years old. I was (and always had been), as my doctors called it, "grossly underweight" due to a combined mineral deficiency and a speedy metabolism. When I arrived at my agency office in Taipei for the first time, the crazy thing was that I wasn't the thinnest girl there. I was five foot, nine inches, and ninety-seven pounds. There were girls from all over the planet, ages spanning more than a decade, and I was *far* from the skinniest person in the room. *Had I found my people?*

To better understand this comment, I think it is important to know that most of my tween years were permeated by hurtful name-calling and atrocious bullying: "Anorexic," "Maybe you should eat a sandwich," "I could wash my clothes on your chest, *flatty*," "Hey, beanpole; twig; scrappy; stix; scrawn-bag; training bra." (Yes, one delightful boy nicknamed me "training bra.") I had heard it all and still do from time to time in the depths of my subconscious thoughts. So my experience in

Taiwan somehow became my acceptance—permission to finally see my "grossly underweight" stature as attractive, even desirable.

I never personally suffered from an eating disorder, but it was rampant in my circles. I did, however, suffer from major body-image conflicts, insurmountable insecurity about my weight and waist size (which was mainly fueled by the weekly weigh-in and measuring sessions by my agency), and I experienced a lot of pressure to conform to really ridiculous and, now knowing, unhealthy guidelines. At sixteen years old, I was offered my first line of cocaine, which was referred to as "the skinny dust" and used more as a dietary aid than your typical recreational drug. I respectfully declined even though the offer came from a mentor and guardian. On this same trip I watched three of my flatmates eat tissue (yes, the kind you blow your nose with) as a meal because "it expands in your stomach and takes away the hunger." These memories are for another book, however. My point is this: Health *can* be subjective, almost like age. "You are only as old as you feel." Well, *you are only as healthy as you feel too*, to some degree. Health can largely be a mindset. A lifestyle. An ongoing effort to be the best version of yourself. It doesn't matter which diet trend you choose to participate in or which workout fad. **You do you!** How do **you** feel? What makes **you** feel good? Where do **you** want to see changes? How would these changes improve the quality of **your** life? I am positive you won't find the answers by eating tissues for dinner or taking up a cocaine habit.

Sorry to be the bearer of bad news, Mama, but there is no little magic pill that will diminish stretch marks or make those thirty pounds disappear. There is no secret sauce that will work for every mama out there either. *Why?* Because we are all different—comprised of almost 7,000,000,000,000,000,000,000,000,000 (also known as seven billion billion billion) unique particles that make us who we are.[2] Wouldn't it be naïve for us to think that *health* could be a one-size-fits-all scenario? Thus, the latter definition became the framework for this book. Soundness, capability, balance. "Holistic" (whole-ness) is a word that surfaced a lot in the stories too. Health, to me, really is about harmony. The **body** needs the **mind** and the **spirit** to function as a well-oiled machine for optimal health.

I knew when researching for this book it was imperative to find the right people, the ideal tribe, to cover all the schools of thought around health (because as you can see, it is incredibly diverse). You will hear from Western medicine doctors, Chinese medicine doctors, naturopathic doctors, nutritionists, educators, fitness professionals, personal trainers, Pilates instructors, registered nurses, wellness coaches, and many experienced mamas. This is not a "how-to" book on getting healthy or your typical one-sided guide to "this" diet or "that" workout routine. The stories shared over the next three hundred pages are the authentic journeys of mamas who have been on all sides of health.

The sections of this book are broken into the sections of soundness. We focus first on BODY and cover topics including nutrition, fitness, nourishing ourselves and our children, pelvic floor health, body image, and holistic postpartum recovery. Our physical body changes a lot when we have children. Whether or not you have stretch marks, extra weight, a spare tire, mom-tum, pelvic floor challenges, or you look like a bodybuilder, it is important to realize that you are a different person than you were before you had a child. I want to encourage you to embrace *Her*, this new version of yourself. Any time you feel down about your body remember the warrior that you are. You created and housed human life inside that magical body, Mama. I think it is also really important to be gentle and kind to ourselves. Please remember that health is not defined by our weight or the perkiness of our breasts. It took me a while to get used to the new me. After almost twenty years in the modeling industry, twenty years of having my measurements taken regularly and being told what to eat and how to look, twenty years of seeing photoshopped abs and makeup highlights accentuating my calf muscles in photos, to look in the mirror and see an extra forty pounds and dimpled skin was an adjustment. Our worth is not defined by our appearance. Our children and those who matter will see our battle scars as beauty marks. Love is so much deeper than skin, and the most important love you can have is love for yourself. Your whole self. Love yourself for just the way you are.

In the second section, we dive into topics of the MIND—*this* is more my *jam*. I have always been obsessed with all things psychological and find the human brain and its marvelous ways quite fascinating. We speak a lot about mental health, postpartum depression, dealing with a sick child, surrendering, grief, loss, mindset, and personal growth. This section became so important because I have yet to meet a mother who hasn't come up against some self-doubt or questioning. When you become a mother, your life changes so drastically, and not just physically and socially, but internally as well. It is especially important that we speak about the internal changes as every single mama has experienced this bittersweet roller coaster—stepping into her new everything (body, identity, schedule, social life, and more) while still trying to hang onto who she once was and trying to find that happy medium between the two. One of my biggest struggles as a new mom was saying good-bye to the lifestyle and freedom I once had. I eventually embraced the extra roll on my belly and the sciatic nerve damage, the stubborn hemorrhoids, and the minor pelvic floor prolapse. I did, however, have a difficult time managing the isolation, feeling like I was trapped every moment of every day like I couldn't shower or run an errand without a human hip attachment. Just like our body needs nourishment and exercise to stay sound, so does our mind. We must feed our mind healthy thoughts and keep it active.

Lastly is the SPIRIT section where we meet our soulful warriors, some of whom were and still are in the thick of their fertility journeys. We explore how they used spiritual practices to overcome obstacles. It took me many years of personal development to discover my spiritual side and to realize it's not all voodoo and witchcraft. I do not actively practice religion or go to church, but I consider myself a student of the Universe. I believe in fate and the notion that everything happens for a reason, by divine intervention. The concept of spirituality is quickly becoming more conventional and intertwined with mental health. The understanding is that practices like meditation, visualization, and affirmations can be extremely helpful in calming the mind, and the simple act of deep breathing can improve your overall health. The women in this section very eloquently share their journeys with us. These are real stories, shared by the women who experienced them. Like all our *You've Got This, Mama* books, this one is also incredibly raw and authentic.

What I have personally learned about *health* is that it is fluid and ever changing. I don't just mean the data either. Health is volatile—it can turn at any minute, in any direction. We must collectively work with all our faculties to keep ourselves sound. I write these words from an interesting place in my life. My mother, who is the average age a mother of a thirty-something-year-old would be, recently fell and broke her pelvis, but not because she is frail and old. She is in impeccable health. She has good bones and nutrition, and she takes naturopathic supplements. She tripped over our family dog in the kitchen and fell, and three seconds later, her entire world changed. The reason this seemingly undramatic event affected me so is because it put a thing or two into perspective. We can be healthy, but we are not invincible. Life is fragile and volatile. We must be cautious without being fearful. We must exercise our capabilities to maintain optimal health. There is no blanket remedy for anything. There is embracing change as it comes at you. There is nourishing your body, mind, and spirit with the fuels that best serve **you** as an individual. There is loving yourself and being kind to the mother, the partner, the daughter, and the woman you are, and there is living this one life you've got as best you can. There is remembering that wherever you are in your health and wellness journey, **you've got this, Mama!**

Section One

BODY

FEATURING

Daphne Kostova

Jennifer Kaley Smits

Stephanie Moody

Naomi Haupt

Melissa Smith

Tara Butterwick

Hillary Dinning

OPENING COMMENTARY BY

Sabrina Greer

The body is defined as the physical structure of a person or an animal, including the bones, flesh, and organs. If this definition is so, *our body is just a pile of flesh used for housing organs and bones*, why do we put so much pressure and drama on the way it *looks*? As mothers, we have experienced the miracles that the old bag of bones is capable of creating. Yet we have so many negative thoughts and feelings about our bodies. *What is this spare tire? I'm disgusting. I wish I could still fit into [fill in the blank with a piece of clothing from a decade ago].* Our bodies, much like our minds, our responsibilities, and our lives are meant to change after children. Change is inevitable, but we often resist it.

Working in the modeling industry for nearly two decades made me both detached from and acutely aware of my body. One event that will forever stand out as an eye-opener for me was the first time I went to Milan, Italy, on a modeling contract. I was eighteen years old, before the age of cell phones, GPS, and Instagram filters, in the fashion capital of the world. I was (and still am) what I like to call *directionally challenged*. But I was okay because I had a map. Yup, you read that right: a good ol' fashioned, paper-folding map. I had sixteen castings that day. If you don't know what a casting is, think of it as the equivalent of an audition for an actor, but there is no acting and you are judged entirely on the way you look. On that blessed day I had sixteen of them. Translation—I had to navigate the transit system of an unfamiliar city while in high heels with a heavy portfolio bag and my directional deficiency. This experience also meant sixteen people (or groups of people), speaking in foreign languages, needed to see me in my bikini, measure my body parts, and *judge* every ounce of my flesh. I hadn't eaten that day, a trick my agent taught me to "keep my stomach flat," so I felt faint and ill to boot. Lucky for me, one building housed four of the sixteen castings. *Phew, less traveling!*

When I arrived at said building, I ran into my stunning German-Greek flatmate who happened to speak seven languages. I was excited because all the clients spoke languages I could not understand, and now I had a translator, someone who could share their comments. Casting One went well, I thought. They poked and prodded but seemed content with my structure. Casting Two had literal eye-rolls and hand gestures that needed no translation. They did not like what they saw. Casting Three: Other than the large man who smelled my hair, the rest of the clients seemed less creepy and ready to hire me. Lastly was Casting Four—not what I would call a confidence builder, but you can't be everyone's cup of tea, right?

During a tram-ride reunion with my flatmate post-casting frenzy, I asked her what was said about me. Casting Two had said something along the lines of "She needs to eat a sandwich, that scrappy chicken." Casting Four said I was far too "fat" for their flavor. Why was this such a pivotal moment in my career and life? I realized in that moment that I would never be vanilla, a flavor that everyone likes. I would never be Play-Doh squeezed into the proverbial mold people wanted me to fit in. I realized that what others thought of me was none of my business, and I no longer cared about what *they* thought. What mattered was how *I* felt about myself. NEXT!

I have kept this life lesson close, and it has served me well in the massive changes motherhood has brought to my body. We need to stop right now: stop putting pressure on ourselves to "bounce back" or try to fit into the skin we have already shed. We have to stop comparing ourselves to others. We have to stop hating and judging the reflection in the mirror, and we HAVE to stop giving even a single fuck about what anybody else thinks. You are a freaking miracle. Your body created, grew, and fed a human life. Repeat after me: "I am a miracle!"

I remember after my first son was born, at four weeks' postpartum, I was desperate to get back to the gym. My inner demented model programming told me, *that's what we do*. During childbirth, I received an episiotomy, had second-degree tearing, got four stitches, and had a completely open diastasis recti. Did I mention my son was ten pounds? My doctors and midwives strongly opposed this idea of mine to return to the gym. My midwife said something that imprinted on my mind. She said, "Sabrina, you have an open wound inside your body the size of that baby (so rather large). You need at least as much time to heal as it took to create this life." This advice has stuck with me. She was not in any way demonizing exercise, but she was reminding me that we need to be gentle with our bodies in the same way we would nurture a broken bone or flesh wound.

I tell you this story with the hope that it will inspire you to be even a little bit kinder to yourself—to your body, your mind, and your spirit. Be gentle physically and allow for healing. Go easy on the negative self-talk and remind yourself what your body has been through. Be grateful for the gift and remember that your flesh does not define you. Be you, Mama, because you are beautiful just the way you are.

Go for what
empowers you
and you'll
empower others.

~Daphne Kostova
@daphne_wellness

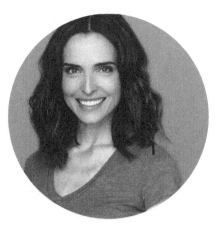

Daphne Kostova

Daphne Kostova, CNP, is a Toronto-based holistic nutritionist. Daphne was born in Bulgaria and has fond memories of spending her summer vacations in her baba's (*grandma* in Bulgarian) organic fruit and vegetable garden. Her favorite childhood memory is sitting up high on the cherry tree branches, carelessly daydreaming and enjoying the fresh, ripe fruit. Her baba lived an active, happy life, nourished by what her garden brought her, all the way to one hundred years old. She taught Daphne many valuable life lessons throughout their time together.

Daphne moved to Toronto with her husband in her early twenties. She worked as a model and an actress for the next fifteen years, taking short breaks in between to have her children. Daphne is a devoted (and very proud) mother of Boris, eleven years old, and Laura, five years old. She loves making natural skincare products (she has her own brand called **Daphne's Apothecary**) and enjoys digging into everything related to clinical functional nutrition and supplementation.

Whenever she is not working with clients toward their best health or delving into the latest news on nutrition and natural skincare formulas, Daphne loves hiking in the forest or biking on trails with her family. Nutrition, fitness, natural cosmetics, writing, and economics (she also holds an iB.B.A.) are some of her biggest interests and pleasures.

Daphne believes being present and open to the new challenges life brings is a freeing experience with incredible benefits along the way.

Ⓦ dkwellnesssolutions.com

f Dk wellness solutions

Ⓘ @dk.wellness.solutions

~ To my mom, Zorka: You are the best teacher of unconditional love. To my godmom, Boriana K. and my children's godmom, Mira K.: You are my forever teachers. To Marlene: Thank you for being a part of my birth stories; thank you for being family. You are forever embedded in my most grateful thoughts and prayers. Grateful for all of you!

One

LOVE OR FEAR
Daphne Kostova

*"The point of power is always in the present
moment. This is where we begin to make
changes."*
~Louise L. Hay

I went for a run tonight. Typically, I love running, especially during early
mornings when it is quiet in the big city. Mornings are a lot cooler during
the hot summer days, and the run feels more private in my neighborhood. Over the last fifteen years, running has become my secret weapon
and sidekick, helping me de-stress from the day-to-day pressures of life.
Tonight was no different. Tonight I needed to hit the sidewalk. I saw my
husband's car pull up in the driveway. As we passed each other at our
front entrance, I asked if he could watch the kids while I went for a run.
I felt exhausted both physically and emotionally, but I knew running
would help me. It always did. As much as I watched the passersby to
avoid bumping into them, my experience was mainly with myself. I could
lose myself in my run. I needed to visualize whatever was happening in
my mind, and running helped me do this. It grounded me and helped

me clear my mind and emotions and always provided me with solutions on moving forward in any situation. When I was pregnant with my children, I engaged in regular exercise such as running (during my first trimester) and swimming (second and third trimesters) to not only stay healthy and ensure a healthy pregnancy and delivery but also to numb any anxiety I had regarding their upcoming births. Now, however, I was running for myself. Tonight I needed to let go of the fear that *I wasn't enough as a mom*, and moreover, the fear surrounding my mom's cancer diagnosis. I was scared of losing her, and I needed to release that fear, implement some changes, and turn things around. I needed to find a way to be proactive. *This* was exactly how I had prepared myself for my milestone of becoming a mother and delivering my two beautiful babies. I knew *this* was exactly how I would gain clarity on *what* to do and *how* to be most helpful with my mom's diagnosis.

As I continued to run through the city, my mind flashed back to when I gave birth to my children. I realized that everything about my birth plans stemmed from a place of love, and that's why I felt empowered and fearless no matter the uncertainty that surrounded them. I was focused on their health (and my health too!). I wanted them to be born with healthy gut flora, which meant having a natural home birth, and I wanted to breastfeed them for two years each since breast milk is known to be the most beneficial food to help boost their immunity according to the baby books and literature I read (side note: Fed is best, no matter which route you go!). I remember feeling anxious while I was in labor. I remember feeling scared, but everything went as planned. My boy was born in our first home with just my husband, Victor, and me, and our midwife, Marlene. He was perfect (and born on his due date!). I remember our cherry tree blooming that very day as well. It was picture-perfect; I still warm up, letting happiness and love wash over me as I beam with pride just thinking about my first birth experience. My midwife placed him on my belly, and just like it's written in the parenting books, he climbed upward, found his milk, and started breastfeeding. He breastfed for three years.

It all sounds so easy, but it wasn't always like that! I had mastitis a couple times. At one point my son was three months old, and I had already returned to work as I had no maternity leave. Having had a painkiller-free birth, I knew what pain was and I knew I could tolerate it. However, the pain that accompanies birthing is also something you mentally prepare yourself for over nine months, and your body releases endorphins to soothe the pain. Mastitis came about unexpectedly, and along with it came a 40°C fever. I felt like my eyeballs were on fire due to the fever caused by the infection. Breastfeeding during mastitis is highly recommended so that the milk ducts get emptied, thus providing you with some relief. The funny part is that you can breastfeed in every possible position in an attempt to relieve the pain and unclog the exact duct that clogged this way in the first place!

I also remember getting sick and almost losing my milk when my son was fifteen months old. It took a lot of effort to maintain it, and I wanted to ensure he was breastfed as he was due for a small surgery at eighteen months. After the surgery was complete, my son was given back to me all red and swollen and crying inconsolably. I knew something was wrong. A mother's instincts never lie. I felt like the solution was for me to breastfeed him, and so I did. Breastfeeding calmed him right away, his allergic reaction diminished significantly (thanks also to him being given a small dose of Benadryl), and his breathing returned to normal. The explanation we were given by the medical team was that "he must have been allergic to one of the meds in anesthesia." I didn't know this fact back then, but anesthesia consists of many different medications (that the doctors that day did not wish to name, nor could our medical team identify exactly which medication induced my son's allergic reaction). Additionally, anesthesia causes dysbiosis and, in this case, breastfeeding was the best way to get the healthy bacteria into my son so his gastro-intestinal system could return to a healthy balance with the pathogens (the bad bacteria) as well as simultaneously soothe his distress. I wasn't a holistic nutritionist back then. It wasn't my nutritional knowledge that helped, rather *it was my plain, primal instinct as a mother that helped me to help my son.* Boris Max recovered quickly post surgery.

My daughter was born at home too, six years later, with the same crew—Victor, Marlene, and me. I often wonder how people perceive the home-birth experience if they haven't done it themselves. Home birth is not glamorous! I spent most of my birthing time walking around my home or sitting on the toilet or on the birthing stool. Lying on the bed was the last thing I wanted to do because, well, try lying down with pos-terior babies (their backs are pushing your back). It causes excruciating back pain, and for me, it was more painful than the actual birth itself. However, I do not remember most of the process. I remember vividly seeing my babies for the first time. I remember hearing my son's loud cry and feeling his strong grip on my hand. I remember Marlene calling him a "hurricane baby," which I thought was such a cool metaphor for his personality! Boris Max lives up to it every day. When Laura Bella was born, Marlene said she caught her in her arms like a "sweet chocolate bar." Laura had a soft and gentle voice, and her whole energy was that of grace—the trace of an old soul being born. The first impression she made stayed and became a part of her personality. I let out a sigh of contentment and smiled from cheek to cheek as I continued my run. I felt like I was so close to reaching the clarity I was seeking regarding my mom's diagnosis, and all I needed to do was trust my instincts. I glanced up at the sky, which was a beautiful shade of orange, pink, and blue. The sun was setting and, juxtaposed against the city lights and skyscrapers, it looked beautiful.

I have always felt that becoming a mom is a great honor and a work of art. We can give ourselves the gift and privilege of being loving, caring, and responsible for another human's well-being, and we don't even need a license or permission slip. Similar to how we spend hours and months learning how to drive a car, we should put the same (if not more) effort and gusto into researching and preparing for motherhood! That's not all. I learned as I was raising my own children that I had to nourish my relationship with my mother. I needed to repair my relationship with her and make an effort to be closer to her. It all comes full circle, and I had to learn to fully respect everyone involved.

I continued reflecting on my relationship with my mother. It's one of those nights. It's one of those runs where I confronted all my fears for a change. I had had a hard time being my parents' child growing up. My parents are amazing people; they are loving, caring, and very giving. They became parents in their late thirties (very late for their time) because my mom waited to finish her professional degrees. As a result, I felt the generational gap immensely in my youth. I was raised in Plovdiv, Bulgaria, and I immigrated to Canada with my partner in my early twenties. My move created an even greater distance between my parents and me. Each year, as I delve further into motherhood, I have a deeper understanding of what it must have cost my mom to be the most amazing mom to me, to raise me the way she did, and to love me the way she did. Understanding and appreciating my mother more and more with time brings peace and warmth to my soul. We were different individuals—she was calm, centered, introverted, and very intelligent. As a kid, I was extroverted, quick to decide, and impatient. I had immense pride every time I stepped into my hometown university where she was a professor of organic analytical chemistry. I feel so grateful to have her as a mom. What a privilege to be raised by one of the most intelligent women of her time—a woman of strength, elegance, quiet grace, and beauty! I felt clear-headed. I felt reassured. I felt much calmer than when I started the run an hour previously. I was finally at the front of my house, bending forward, placing my hands on my knees, and catching my breath before I headed into the beautiful yet chaotic mess that is my life and motherhood.

Tonight I needed to go for a run to put things back into perspective and reframe my perception of motherhood. Yes, I have great birthing stories, and I am proud of my children and so grateful and happy to be their mom. They are truly amazing, and, if at all possible, a bigger challenge for me than I was for my own mom. I attended family therapy sessions with my kids in order to gain a better understanding of how to best relate to their needs. What followed were months of pillow fights with my eldest (who was eight at the time). As an eight-year-old kid, it was his way of relating to me through play and an incredible tool to make us giggle and continue our day with ease. Another amazing tool I discovered is simply devoting twenty minutes a day with my child(ren) and doing exactly what they want: soccer, video games, or a trampoline. As long as the activity is their decision and we do it together, it is their way to relate to us best and to feel understood.

Tonight I also needed to run to gain some clarity. My mom was diagnosed with cancer a year ago. She believes her disease stems from spending years in a chemistry research lab without proper protection against toxic chemical exposure. It is the only explanation I have as I know how well my mother fed us and taught us to respect our bodies through proper nutrition and movement. The sour and bitter stench at her workplace (located next to the university labs) is one that is forever embedded in my senses. We cannot change the past, however, but we can change our future and make it better. Since my mom chose chemotherapy as her ammunition against cancer, I have pulled up my sleeves and researched the best sources of information to provide her with clinical nutrition and supplementation to keep her strong and healthy during treatments. I do believe my mom needs my help in her battle against cancer, but more than anything else, she needs my love and understanding. We can't let fear creep in.

Tonight I went for a run to process everything: motherhood, my childhood, the relationship we have with our children, and the relationship we have with our parents, especially our mothers. Yes, it matters how we care for our babies, what we feed them, how we supplement their nutrition. Yes, it was my plan to have a natural birth. But even if natural birth wasn't the case, I would have still given breastfeeding a try to ensure healthy gut flora and steady brain development for my babies. And if I wasn't able to breastfeed, that's okay too. There are some quality natural formula blends and supplements to provide babies with nutrients and nourishment, and a good, healthy lifestyle makes all the difference. What I once thought was the most important thing was only a piece of the puzzle. All I am saying, Mama, is one unachieved goal does not mean that you crash and burn. There is always room to be flexible and make things work beautifully as long as it works for you and your family! I believe my kids need great nutrition and supplementation hands down, but feeling love for my son and showing him that love sometimes means letting him eat a small bag of chips and watching the joy on his face as he devours the bag (side note: After reading some of my books, he now chooses chips from natural food stores when available). I used to be so stubborn about my children consuming junk food, but I get it now. To my son, my action of letting him have a bag of chips means love and understanding from my part as his mother. So I give in sometimes. He needs my love more than anything, and he will learn all about nutrition soon enough! I sometimes find him sitting in front of my nutrition/well-being library at home reading my books. He asks me questions about them. Flexibility and curiosity at its best!

Something else my journey as a woman and a mother has taught me is how to feel my way into life. As humans, I believe we only feel two main emotions: fear and love. Every other emotion stems from these two basal emotions. When we approach a situation with love, we choose to be open, we are willing to learn and educate ourselves, and we may even embrace another perspective or way of life for we have the right to change our mind. We choose to forgive our own mistakes and those of others too. We accept ourselves and those around us—imperfections, quirks, and all! Fear works the opposite way. It weaves its spell on us, trapping us in our insecurities. It is unforgiving and harsh, and its grasp on us can be so tight that it can dim our light and life force. It can even make us ill.

As mothers, daughters, and most of all, as women, we tend to internalize everything and absorb the stressors around us—the energy of each situation and each person, without question or a second thought. We do so because we are born nurturers who take care of the world around us. A certain amount of stress is a normal part of daily life. However, when stress becomes overwhelming and prolonged, the risks for health problems increase. Long-term stress increases the risk of adrenal imbalance, headaches, gastrointestinal problems, and a weakened immune system. I have felt the effects of stress on my adrenals, and I have learned how to help myself and others through remedies and lifestyle adjustments, some of which are listed below:

- Sleep, rest, and moderate exercise are your best friends. Avoid caffeine, sugar and artificial sweeteners, and processed carbs for a while. See how you feel if you go gluten free and without starch for some time.

- Avoid hydrogenated oils and processed foods.

- Raw nuts and seeds (almonds, walnuts, sunflower seeds, pumpkin seeds, flax seeds, etc.), avocado, cruciferous vegetables (broccoli, cauliflower, brussels sprouts, etc.), fatty fish (wild-caught Atlantic salmon), organic poultry, bone broth, Himalayan salt, fermented foods, and seaweed are great choices to add to your diet.

- Great support supplements are vitamins C, B complex, magnesium, a potent multivitamin and adaptogenic herbal blend, licorice root, fish oil, and selenium. Calming essential oils such as rose and lavender oil are great tools too. However, I strongly recommend you speak to a holistic nutritionist so your individual profile and needs are taken into consideration.

My advice is to pick a few things that you know will work for you and your family and adhere to them as your nonnegotiable mental, emotional, and physical deep clean. Keep love and understanding at the forefront of your healing practice as a mother, a daughter, a wife, and a woman. My own mental health depends on these techniques, and putting in the work consistently such as going for a run or meditating helps me navigate through life as a mom and a busy professional. I truly believe in the power of having a community, asking for help, and researching the heck out of something when I am not sure what else to do. Choose to live from a place of love, not fear. This choice alone will empower you to live a healthy life that nourishes you and your family—mind, body, and soul. Choose love and curiosity, openness and acceptance, and the perspective that comes with them. It is a journey of constant learning.

Health and happiness are about the whole self—body, mind, and soul, and having the right mindset and support system to lean on.

You've got this, healthy Mama!

Every moment spent stressing about being perfect is a moment wasted not being present.

~Jennifer Kaley Smits
@jennkaley

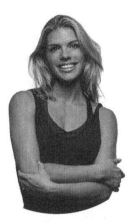

Jennifer Kaley Smits

Scouted by a modeling agency in her teens, Jenny spent the first decade of her adult life modeling and traveling. In her twenties, she decided to take a different path in life. She knew she needed to take care of her body and live a healthier lifestyle.

She enrolled at George Brown College (Toronto) in its university program where she completed a culinary and nutrition degree and graduated with Honors.

Having struggled with body image most of her life, she desired to help others live a healthy and balanced life: mentally, socially, physically, and spiritually.

Jenny flew to the Bahamas and took an intensive yoga teacher training course. She found yoga to be an amazing tool to center her and help find balance in her life.

After living in her East Coast home for a couple of years, she continued on her journey of health and fitness. Jenny attended a conference on eating disorders and had the privilege of visiting one of the best inpatient treatment centers in America. This visit made her more determined to help others with health and fitness. She returned to Toronto and added a certification in Pilates to her résumé.

While in Toronto, Jenny met and married the love of her life, and they now have a beautiful two-year-old son. Nothing prepared Jenny for the journey of motherhood. However, the sheer joy of spending time with her little guy has been her greatest love and life accomplishment.

 jennkaley.ca

@jennkaley

~ This chapter is dedicated to my best friend, my husband, who during this journey of motherhood stood by my side in the good times and the bad. He has been my strength when I thought I could not take another step. I am so grateful for our little family.

Two

IT'S ALL MOMENTARY
Jennifer Kaley Smits

*"There's no way to be a perfect mother, and a
million ways to be a good one."*
~Jill Churchill

I can honestly say my childhood was really great! I had a loving mother, father, and older brother. We loved one another and enjoyed life together. We had family dinners every night. Friday night was always *treat* night when we had pizza or hamburgers. I always felt very secure and safe. I have memories of our home being very welcoming, and my brother and I had many of our friends stay for sleepovers and shared meals. My dad often said our home had the "vacuum effect"—once someone came for a visit, they were sucked in and always returned. This fact is true even today. I honestly thought my parents never fought, all my needs were met, and my life was blessed. My memories are also full of family traditions, delicious home-cooked meals, and fun family vacations. Our summer days were the best. There was swimming and boating with family and the many friends who were always welcomed at our family cottage.

High school is when things began to change. I imagine like any preteen girl budding into womanhood, I started questioning my body. My brother and I weren't as close as we once were when we were children, and social pressures began to shatter my perfect world. Like many of the girls at school, I started judging my worth by the shape and size of my body. Magazines and television made thin look so very appealing. I was in competitive dance growing up and my physique was naturally thin, but suddenly I felt fat. My eating patterns changed yet went unnoticed by others. I guess my dancer bod masked it well. At first, my obsession with food did not raise red flags until . . . I became interested in modeling. I signed with a local agency and started doing some modeling, and I was working toward entering a modeling competition in Toronto. I developed what I know now was an eating disorder—but not the kind where you eat chocolate cake and then spend hours purging in the bathroom, not the kind where you eat tissue paper or stop eating altogether. Mine was entirely psychological. I counted calories and had all-consuming thoughts of what was going into my body. It was an exhausting and stressful time. This type of eating disorder is now recognized in the Diagnostic and Statistical Manual of Mental Disorders as Eating Disorder Not Otherwise Specified (EDNOS).

At seventeen years old I was very excited to travel to the modeling competition in Toronto. Did I want to embark on this career path, or did I need validation for all my *hard* work? I was scouted by a well-known modeling agency. Perhaps you've heard of it? Ford Models. Shortly after that whirlwind, I moved to Toronto. I quickly immersed myself in all things modeling, affirming my previous obsessions. Body image, weight control, and dieting surrounded me and quickly became part of my daily routine. My twenties focused on watching my weight, and I adopted the belief system of good food/bad food. My days and moments were filled with all-consuming thoughts about *what* I was eating, *when* I was eating, and *how* I could find time to get to the gym.

After having a career in modeling for over a decade, I decided to pursue a different path, a healthier path. I had always enjoyed exercising and healthy eating. I decided I wanted to have a career helping others do what I loved. I wanted to further my education so I could educate others on optimal health. Still anchored in the grand metropolis of Toronto, Ontario, I enrolled myself in a culinary nutrition program at George Brown College and graduated a few years later as a certified nutritionist and chef. Learning about the power of food as fuel and medicine was an incredibly empowering experience. Understanding that *fat* was not the devil and how to appropriately incorporate it into a balanced diet blew my mind.

I became obsessed with education. I became a sponge, hungry for knowledge, soaking it all in. I also pursued my personal training certification, my yoga instructor training, and my Pilates instructor certification so I could take on clients from a holistic approach, customizing their programs with fitness, nutrition, mental health, and breath work. Additionally, I had the privilege of attending a conference called *Hungry for Hope* where I became more knowledgeable about eating disorders and healthy eating. I had the opportunity to visit a leading inpatient treatment center to learn from their nutritionist and experience firsthand what an eating disorder can lead to.

My early thirties felt so aligned. I created and grew a fun career teaching fitness, yoga, and Pilates while helping my clients with nutrition and meal planning. I also found a love: helping my mother with her clients. She is a therapist who specializes in working with people struggling with eating disorders. I created meal plans and recipes for her clients. Life had really come full circle as I could deeply empathize with these young clients, recognizing myself in their sometimes invisible struggle with food.

At this point my boyfriend, Marty, and I had been together for four years and decided to get engaged. Wedding plans quickly commenced as the date was set, the dress was bought, and invitations were mailed to our guests. Two months into the wedding planning process we found out I was pregnant. We were both in shock but super excited at the same time. We decided to move ahead with the wedding as I was so early in my pregnancy and not yet showing.

I had an amazing pregnancy. I was able to maintain my teaching career until my third trimester and stayed active throughout. I went into labor with full confidence that I would have no complications and my baby would just pop out. I mean, I was a fitness instructor and taught yoga. *How hard could it be?* My midwife felt I was a prime candidate for a natural birth. I was happy to try unless there were severe complications. Looking back I realize I did not give myself the grace to be flexible. I did not prepare myself for the unknowns that accompany childbirth. Giving birth is our first experience as a mother—we learn to let go and do what's right for our babies.

My labor was thirty-eight exhausting hours, and I had multiple complications. It turned out that my baby had a short umbilical cord and was struggling to come down the birth canal. I was rushed in for a cesarean section with tears streaming down my face and full of fear that my baby would not survive. After being fully prepped for surgery, the doctor told me there was a ***change*** in plans. I was getting an episiotomy and I had to push. After what seemed like forever, I pushed and my baby boy came out. He was immediately placed on my chest. I was filled with love and fear all at once, like most new, first-time mothers, I imagine. I also felt mostly relieved that my baby's birth journey was over, and he was now safe and snug in my arms.

In that moment, Nate and I began our story. My journey to motherhood began at conception, but our life together and figuring out how to survive outside the coziness of Mama's belly were not at all going as I had planned. The first four months as a new mama were filled with questions, anxiety, and sleepless nights. I started missing my old life and felt extremely guilty for it. I was determined to do everything perfectly, breastfeeding and all. I have never been great at accepting help from anyone other than my mom and dad, and they were two thousand miles away on the east coast. They came as often as they could, but this little guy was solely my responsibility, and I wanted so badly to do everything right. If I were to really SUCCEED at anything in life, I wanted it to be motherhood—being a good mom to my boy.

I would look in the mirror and feel betrayed by my body, however. *How did I, the fitness instructor, put on fifty-two pounds?* All these questions went through my mind daily: *How come I wasn't bouncing back so quickly? Didn't the weight just fall off when you were breastfeeding? Why wasn't I healing quickly enough to get back in the gym?* I would look at other new moms and wonder how they did it. They looked so put together and content. They were showered and wearing makeup. Their babies had on cute outfits. They seemed so rested and happy. *Was I missing something? I must not be doing this right.* I was sending myself into a crazy spiral of self-defeat.

Nate's first Christmas was when I was truly about to fall apart. I flew back east to be with my family and enjoy the Christmas holidays with everyone. I was hopeful that with my family around and some extra hands I would get out of the sad headspace I was in. Even though I have the most incredible husband and loving supportive family who sincerely wanted to help, I felt I *had* to remain in control of taking care of Nate. He was waking every hour and the sleepless nights were catching up with me.

After I had a small breakdown, my mom, who as I mentioned is a therapist, sat me down and told me she felt I was experiencing postpartum depression. She kindly told me that life doesn't always go as we plan. She encouraged me by saying that it was okay if being a mom wasn't going as I had imagined. I found it so difficult that things were not as I had planned. Breastfeeding was tough, he wasn't latching well, and he wasn't sleeping. Maybe my little guy and I would just figure it out together.

January was a real time of growth for me as a mom. I slowly learned to let go of control and began allowing for help in all areas of my life. We hired a sleep consultant. Nate began to sleep and nap, and thus, I felt rested and clear-headed. Being a mom became easier for me, and Nate and I were more comfortable with our daily patterns. But . . . I still had all my baby weight and felt very uncomfortable in my skin. I was back teaching fitness classes and felt like I was under a microscope of judgment, which produced major feelings of shame.

In this area, I still felt deflated, like all my former strength was gone. What I used to look like was a distant memory. My pre-baby body was strong with defined and toned muscles. I walked around with confidence knowing I was physically strong. Looking in the mirror after baby, I didn't recognize my reflection. I was soft, had no muscle tone, and had all sorts of sagging skin. I had rounded shoulders from breastfeeding. I felt lifeless. I was nurturing a complete and total pity party.

I stood by the mirror with tears in my eyes and remembered a conversation with my best girlfriend, Sabrina, before I had Nate. She shared her mantra with me about raising her three boys. "All things are temporary: the good and the bad. It's all momentary." It was at that moment I made a decision. This IS all momentary. Every moment spent stressing about being perfect is a moment wasted not being present with my biggest accomplishment: my son.

I changed my perspective about my new life. I began to thank my body for creating life. I began to thank myself for getting up every day and being a **good** mom to Nate (not a perfect one). I stopped striving for perfection. I began to let others help me. I became more patient with myself and my body. I got back to the gym and started eating healthfully. I stopped wallowing in self-pity. I began to feel confident, not because I had toned, strong muscles, but because I had found who I was truly meant to be in this journey: Nate's mom.

Our society places so much pressure on mothers to be PERFECT. Facebook mom groups are full of mom-shaming, judgment, and ridicule. Social media is full of Pinterest-worthy photographs of new moms who have their pre-baby bodies back at six weeks' postpartum. Instagram shows off beautifully curated, professional images of rested mamas holding their well-dressed infants. But it is the highlight reel, the staged and filtered version. It is an evolved version of the societal pressure I've always felt, and I guess on some level or another, it will always exist.

My greatest lesson on this journey to becoming Nate's mom that I want to share in hopes of inspiring you is this: It is all momentary. Life is about how you spend every moment that you are graced with. If we think of moments as being numbered, like currency, how would we spend them? Would we waste them worrying about what other people think? Would we spend them in our own head counting calories? I don't know about you, but I don't have enough moments to waste on things that do not serve me or my family. Time is too precious. I try every day to be balanced physically, mentally, socially, and spiritually. It doesn't always happen, but in the moments where things seem to be falling apart, I have learned to give myself space to embrace the imperfections. I have learned to give myself grace. Having Nate has made me want to better myself so I can be a good mom to him. It has made me want to create special moments with him and my husband, to live a life that truly honors my soul and lights me up—a life that makes me feel like I have so much to give to the world, starting with my little boy. He is, and will forever be, my greatest teacher and gift.

To the mamas who are struggling with the reflection in the mirror, please know that you are beautiful. Your body created another beautiful life. That is no easy feat. So, Mama, when you look in that mirror today, let your eyes linger for a moment on your face, your body, your belly, your every curve and scar. This is you, all of you, in all your beautiful, ferocious glory. As you look at yourself with admiration, kindness, and love, remember to give yourself grace, especially when it all feels impossible. And most of all, **remember that everything is momentary.**

There is so much goodness in slowing down and sitting still.

-Stephanie Moody
@drstephaniemoody

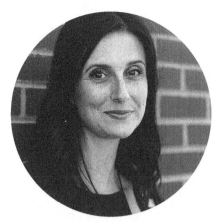

Dr. Stephanie Moody, DC

Dr. Stephanie Moody is a mother of two and a chiropractor with a focus in pre- and postnatal women's health and pediatric wellness. She has dedicated her career to supporting women and their families throughout pregnancy, postpartum, and all stages of motherhood.

After becoming a mother herself, she saw a gap in the care provided for women and families after baby arrives. Even as a women's health professional, she felt lost in all the information and disconnected from her body and herself. It is her goal to set a new standard for postpartum care so that women feel connected in motherhood.

Stephanie practices and teaches workshops in Calgary, Alberta, where she combines gentle manual therapy, functional movement, and education to help women connect to their body and themselves. She believes in the importance of community and supporting one another in motherhood. Stephanie loves bringing together trusted resources in the community and quality, researched information on everything related to movement, motherhood, health, and nutrition.

Ⓦ drstephaniemoody.com

Ⓘ @drstephaniemoody

~ To my amazing parents for whom I am beyond grateful. Mom, for the unconditional love and support and teaching us to see the best in everyone and everything. Dad, I miss you more than words can say. You taught me so much: to not let fear ever hold you back from your dreams or this life and to just go for it. I love you and thank you.

Three

HEALING IN MOTHERHOOD
Dr. Stephanie Moody

"The well-being of mothers is the fabric from which the cloth of the future of our society is made."

~Dr. Oscar Serrallach

Exhausted, anxious, and completely depleted is how I felt after the birth of my second child. These feelings hit me like an overwhelming wall when he was eight weeks old. I expected, of course, to be tired with two small children, but I felt like my body and my brain were crashing. Emotionally, I was angry all the time and snapped at the smallest things I knew I actually didn't care about. I resented my husband because it felt like the load was much heavier on me than him. It was *me* they needed and wanted in the night; it was *my* body that had changed so much; it was *me* who had a pelvic organ prolapse after my first. I took out the anger on my husband even though he is an amazing dad and man. I snapped at him, and I snapped at my kids. The guilt experienced after these episodes was intense—guilt for acting that way, guilt for feeling like I was not doing enough in my career, and guilt for failing as a mother. Even the term self-care was overwhelming; it felt like one more thing I wasn't doing right. I kept telling myself, *it's fine, I'm fine* because I knew I had so much to be grateful for. I had two healthy, beautiful little ones, a loving husband, and the life I wanted and had created. *So why was I so anxious, irritable, and overwhelmed by everything?* I know that this conversation comes with a lot of privilege, so I kept quiet with others and dismissed my emotions. I ignored the intensity of it all. It was as though I was lost, completely disconnected from myself both physically and emotionally. I felt like an empty shell of myself.

When I look back, I can see now that I didn't give myself the time or space I needed to heal on many levels. My dad passed away when I was pregnant with my eldest. I didn't let myself grieve the way I needed to because I knew that stress could have an impact on my developing baby. I remember being stressed about being stressed and worrying about how it would affect my baby girl. As a result, I shoved that pain inward and really started to disconnect from myself. After her birth, I experienced a grade two pelvic organ prolapse (POP). Pelvic organ prolapse is the descent of the pelvic organs (in my case, the bladder) into the vaginal canal.[1] I was angry at my body; I felt like it had failed somehow. In actuality, my body was screaming at me and giving me just what I needed at that moment to truly heal. It took a long time to listen, but eventually it forced me out of my old patterns of remaining in constant motion for distraction purposes. So I started to slow down. It felt so uncomfortable and foreign because in the stillness, I was forced to face the pain. It was just what I needed. Some energetic schools of thought consider pelvic organ prolapse to be a reflection of our root energy. Our root energy provides a grounding or a stable foundation. It can be disturbed by family death or the lack of support or stability, and it can result in feeling disconnected from the true self.[2] This connection between the emotional and physical self was something I was aware of but hadn't acknowledged as part of my own healing. On a mission to heal my prolapse, I started by addressing the physical symptoms. I remained in a constant state of busyness, which is easy to do as a new mom in this society. In all this *doing*, I had moved farther away from myself, from my body, from my emotions, and ultimately, from me.

Then I had one of those moments that stops you in your tracks. It wasn't some life-altering event. I was in my kitchen, making my little ones another *perfectly* nutritious, organic, grass-fed, whole-foods meal while, of course, not making enough for myself. I was mindlessly shoving chocolate chips in my mouth after not eating breakfast or lunch when I started feeling dizzy as though I may actually pass out. I thought, *What the fuck am I doing?!* It really hit me hard amidst the complete exhaustion, I was putting myself last every single day. For the first time I realized how much I had been neglecting myself, and I was the only one who could change that. Preparing nourishing food for the people I care about is one way I express love, so this was telling. There was no self-love happening at all. That was just a starting point for me—fueling my body. The simple act of making food for myself started to slowly shift everything.

A few months after this realization, I was talking with my then-three-year-old daughter. She was whining at the time, and I asked where her strong words went (we make a game of trying to find them around the house—I found this idea from the *Peaceful Parenting Book*).[3] I then proceeded to say that she needed to ask for what she wanted. I'd probably said it a million times before, but that day I realized that I can say it another ten million times, but if I'm not living it, how can I expect my kids to get it? I had not been asking for what I wanted or needed. In fact, I was just surviving each day. I realized that not only did I need to model this behavior if I wanted my kids to get it, but I needed to do it for myself. I found my voice, my strong words, and I finally started asking for what I wanted out of life.

My children have taught me more than I can ever imagine. I'm quite certain they have already taught me more than I can ever teach them. These beautiful souls have brought such clarity through the chaos. It may happen out of hitting a wall of intense exhaustion, but the demands of raising tiny humans no longer allow you to hide from yourself and can be such an opportunity for growth. They don't need a perfect or ideal "supermom," they just need me. In the process of becoming a mother, I have learned to lean into the discomfort, to let go of the illusion of control, and to be still. Once I was able to sit still and acknowledge these emotions, I could tune out the noise and tune into the innate wisdom that was already there. I could finally listen to what I needed. I could finally just be. It was through this connection to myself that my physical symptoms started healing.

Healing Postpartum

It's been said that when a baby is born, a mother is also born. This saying could not be more true. Becoming a mother forever changes you, and this transition needs to be honored. The focus should not be on bouncing back to your pre-pregnancy state. The truth is that after a baby you will never be the same, but in the most beautiful way. Many traditional cultures view childbirth as the biggest transition in a woman's life and a time for the mother to be mothered. It is a time when a woman is nourished, is encouraged to rest for an extended period, and is supported by her community.

A strong support system for women postpartum, both on a physical and emotional level, is vital but lacking for many in modern society. There needs to be more emphasis on rest and healing instead of getting back to it all as quickly as possible. I think one of the reasons I felt so disconnected from my body and self was because I was ignoring my emotions during my transition—I had the need for rest, and I underestimated the value of asking for help. Once I finally began nourishing myself and creating the space that allowed me to tune into my own needs, my body and physical symptoms started healing. More importantly, these were the things that led me back home to myself.

Nourishment

The nutritional demands to grow and support tiny humans both during pregnancy and postpartum are high. The transition into motherhood is a time when your body is healing from pregnancy and birth. It is a time to replenish the depleted nutrient stores and nourish the new mother. It takes an average of three years after having a baby for a woman to fully restore nutrients within her body.[4] This time estimate does not take into account women who have multiple children closer than three years apart, however. Women who are exclusively breastfeeding also require more calories than at any point in pregnancy. It is definitely not a time to restrict calories in any way, though many women (myself included) find it challenging to simply eat enough whether with a newborn baby or young kids. It takes effort, but fueling our body is a basic human requirement that often gets pushed aside during motherhood. Not eating enough can lead to nutrient depletion, exhaustion, and anxiety, and can put further stress on our adrenals. Eating nourishing food has the power to restore energy, nutrients, heal the body, and balance hormones.

That moment in my kitchen really changed how I viewed making food for myself. Instead of it being yet another task on the to-do list, it became a priority as I made myself a priority. Eating enough and eating well were essential for me to start thriving. Basic, right?! But for me, it was really the first step in listening to what my body needed. Not every day is perfect, but it's not about perfection—it's about taking some effort for yourself rather than living off your kids' leftovers and letting the resentment build. I hesitate to talk about food because it's not about restricting what you eat or following the next food trend, it's about listening to *your* body and remembering that every*body* is different. Food has the power to heal, and if you are simply not consuming enough good food, you cannot heal or thrive.

Early Postpartum

Early postpartum is a sacred time when a mother's body is healing. Rest and nutrition are vital during this period. The tissues are healing, and the body's energy is moving toward recovery. Including quality sources of protein, plenty of fat and warming foods can help replenish and restore. Below are some nourishing and healing tips to boost your health.

At this time when the digestive system is sluggish and the body is using energy to heal, a focus on warm, gently cooked, nutrient-dense foods can help nourish and heal the body. Eating gently cooked veggies instead of only raw foods is both warming and recommended early postpartum. Adding spices such as cinnamon, turmeric, and ginger to meals or smoothies can also be an easy way to add some warmth.

Include plenty of collagen-rich foods such as broth and well-cooked quality meats as the amino acids can help with the healing of tissues.

Fats are vital during this time. Make sure to incorporate plenty into each meal. Ghee, grass-fed butter, nuts and seeds, olive oil, coconut oil, and avocados are just a few examples. Omega 3-rich foods such as eggs, salmon, and grass-fed beef are amazing sources of fat as well.

Decreasing inflammation by decreasing refined, processed foods, sugars, or any foods you may not tolerate well can aid in the healing process.

Most of us know how important hydration is, but adding some warming drinks such as herbal teas like nettle, red raspberry leaf, rooibos, or even sipping on broth can help restore minerals and electrolytes and further replenish the body.

Include traditionally prepared carbohydrates such as soaked and well-cooked oats, rice, quinoa, millet, or grains. Sweet potatoes are another great source. A note when preparing the grains: soak in water overnight at room temperature with a splash of something acidic such as apple cider vinegar or lemon juice. This process helps in ease of digestion and increases the nutrients from these foods.

Soups are an incredible healing food as the broth is nutrient- and collagen-dense, and by adding some hearty veggies and protein, you have a complete warming meal in a cup (since foods you can eat with one hand can be essential some days).

Back-to-Balance Postpartum

Nourishing your body with real food is just as essential beyond the first few months of having a baby, and personally, I found it more challenging to fuel myself as my kids grew older. As I mentioned previously, it can take three years for our nutrient stores to fully replenish after having a baby. For many women, symptoms of depletion and exhaustion start showing up several months or even years later.[5] The first few years with young kiddos can be filled with sleep deprivation, increased stress, and continuous breastfeeding. All these factors play a huge role in your nutritional needs. As mentioned previously, breastfeeding in the first six months requires more energy than the energy needed during pregnancy. If you are not eating enough, the lack of calories sends signals to your body that you're in distress, further increasing the stress hormones and leading to complete exhaustion.

Nutrition is even more important if you are experiencing any sort of pelvic floor dysfunction, no matter how many years postpartum you are. What we eat has a direct effect on our tissues' ability to heal. There is also a strong link between our gut health and our pelvic health. Chronic pelvic floor dysfunction has been associated with deficiencies in B1, B6, B12, folic acid, vitamins D and C, magnesium, iron, and zinc.[6] Simply start by making sure you are eating real food and eating enough. Choose organic and local as much as possible. Ensure you are eating plenty of nutrient-dense, collagen-rich foods and healthy fats. Good, quality supplementation can make all the difference in your energy levels as well as amplify your healing process. Yes, it takes a bit of effort and requires you to show up for yourself consistently, but Mama, you are worth that effort and deserve to feel your best.

Creating Space

The transition into motherhood is intense, messy, beautiful, and completely life changing all at the same time. We need space to honor this shift within our lives and within ourselves. There seems to be a badge of honor in the constant *busyness* of our lives—a race to get back to it all as quickly as possible—but there needs to be more value in rest. There is so much goodness in slowing down and sitting still.

Maybe in all the doing is where we start feeling lost and disconnected from ourselves, our needs, and our body. Everyone's needs are so different, but I think we need to give ourselves the time and the grace to just be. I'm not suggesting that as a mother, you can't achieve or accomplish your own goals; I'm actually suggesting quite the opposite. To sit still you turn off the distractions that are in abundance in our society, the autopilot of running around, and tune into what serves you so that you can thrive each day. Slowing down created space for me to simply be, to feel some of the uncomfortable emotions (the busyness was a distraction for me to avoid this), and to get clear on what I want out of this life. Slowing down allowed me to see that everything I needed was already right here. Creating this space by slowing down is what reconnected me back to myself. *This* is where the real healing took place.

So how do you slow down amidst the wild ride of raising children in a world that seems to be spinning faster than ever? For myself, I simplified our life and our schedule. So much of the running around was *not* essential. We now have at least one day where we have no plans, not even grocery shopping or driving anywhere, and it really helps slow things down (the kids love it!). We get outside every day and connect with nature. It felt pretty amazing when I started showing up for myself and letting go of the rest. I felt like I could really be there and be present for myself and my children. I started saying *no* to the things I didn't want to do and even to my kids. Start by getting really clear on your priorities and boundaries. What do you want long term and in the day to day? Make time for those things! They will look different for each of us. There is only one life and there is only one you, so nurture and nourish yourself, Mama. You deserve as much of your love, kindness, attention, and care as you give the world around you. Let go of the rest to create more space for yourself and the life you want. Let go of perfectionism, let go of expectations, let go of anger, let go of guilt, and put yourself first. **You've got this, you really do.**

You can do
it. You can
get there. You
are worth the
process.

~Naomi Haupt
@momshappinessproject

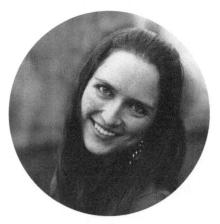

Naomi Haupt

Naomi Haupt was born and raised in Colorado, USA. She takes great interest in people and cultures and has been part of multiple outreach and learning opportunities around the world. An outdoors enthusiast, Naomi trained and worked as a backpacking guide in the Rocky Mountains. She is an artist and musician who participates in various musical ensembles, and she plans to eventually write and record original music. Naomi has always loved writing and has published pieces of poetry, short fiction, and nonfiction. She graduated from Colorado State University in 2010 and married her husband, Charlton, in 2011. Naomi worked for a time as a teacher liaison, helping establish and write curriculum for energy conservation clubs in public schools before transitioning to staying home full time to raise her children.

Through her own experience as a mother and in working with many other moms, Naomi gained a passion for helping moms thrive and be healthy amidst the challenges of raising small children. She founded *The Moms' Happiness Project* in 2017 to provide authentic support and practical strategies and tools for women in the thick of early motherhood.

Naomi is the author of *The Mom's Handbook to Happiness*, a contributing author in *You've Got This, Mama*, and the designer of *Happiness Simplified: The Mom's Organizer*, a daily/weekly/yearly planner made just for moms.

An advocate of women's health and Christian living, Naomi is also a speaker and loves to share about life, God's incredible love, and being a mom.

 themomshappinessproject.com

@momshappinessproject

~ To my parents who first taught me good health habits and laid such a great foundation for my understanding of health today. Thank you!

Four

THE PRINCIPLES OF GOOD MOM-KEEPING
Naomi Haupt

"The secret of change is to focus . . . not on fighting the old, but on building the new."
~Dan Millman

Health as it's understood by a mom, particularly a mom of very young children, is a somewhat broad, vague, guilt-ridden, empowering, life-giving, frustrating, and super important topic. For many of us, both the vision and definition of health and body image get far more complicated after having a baby, and even more so after having multiple babies. All the changes our bodies go through to grow and give birth to a human being are phenomenal when you think about it—I mean, you grew a person. Your body grew a fully formed little person. As incredible as that is, it's not easy on the mom, that's for sure. Muscle changes, vaginal changes, belly changes, hemorrhoids (not cool), breast changes, mental changes . . . it's tough. Beautiful, but tough.

How do we effectively deal with these changes, accept the reality of what our body has gone through, and work toward good health? I use *health* as a general term. Not everyone has the same health goals, and not everyone needs the same health goals. Merriam-Webster defines "health" as *the condition of being sound in body, mind, or spirit.* We're talking about being sound. Being whole. Being healthy. Having what we need to function well, enjoy life, pursue goals, meet responsibilities, and make the most of what we've been given in our bodies, minds, and spirits.

For the purpose of this chapter, we'll be examining physical health, including the area of home cleanliness (trying to keep up with maintaining a healthy home among all the motherhood challenges). To be clear, I am not a health expert or a health professional of any kind. Any concerns you have with your health should be discussed with an appropriate professional. What I'd like to do here, though, is to view health through the lens of motherhood. In other words, how the heck do we, as moms, in all practicality, make positive health changes when our days are already so full and exhausting? It's all well and good to know that we need to be healthy and make good goals and choices for ourselves and our families, but how do we actually implement those choices and work toward those goals in the midst of chaotic days with toddlers, newborns, kids' school schedules, work, relationships, sleep deprivation, and so much more?

Precious Mothers, there are ways. It is doable. It is good. It is really, really important.

Let's take a look.

Perspective

The first and most crucial step to good health as a mom is having a healthy perspective. Mindset, as cliché as it may sound, is super important and paves the way we approach fitness, nutrition, and any other aspect of our well-being. I don't mean a *believe-in-yourself* pep talk (though those can be awfully helpful sometimes) but an entire foundation of perspective. From what I've found in my own experience and from speaking with many other moms, this boils down to a few main pieces:

- **You are you.** You are not anyone else. You don't have to look like anyone else, act like anyone else, or "measure up" to anyone else. This is about *you* being sound, whole, and healthy.

- **Good health changes take place over time.** It's a marathon, not a sprint. Any physical and mental changes that are going to last take time, and as frustrating as that may be sometimes, it's the truth. It's better and far more effective to work with this reality than against it.

- **There is no one "correct" or "best" way to get healthier.** Different things work for different people. Let's face it: Life as a mom of little ones is rarely predictable. We have to find what works for us individually, and it's okay if that changes once, twice, or a hundred times in the process.

Okay, let's get into the practical application. You'll see that I've divided the following into three categories—nutrition, fitness, and household. The goal here is not to tell you what you should be doing but to show you in a real-world way that even as a busy mom, positive health changes are doable and sustainable.

Nutrition

While most of us have goals of some sort or another to change our diet for the better, actually making those changes can be overwhelming. What healthy eating really comes down to is having a lifestyle of good food and drink choices. It's not about a "cold-turkey" dive into some diet we cannot maintain (which may not be good for us anyway), but a piece-by-piece building of habit changes that turn into a bigger, lasting change for the better.

Let's examine a few practicals here. I'm going to use some examples in no particular order. These may or may not be the specific health changes you're going for, but again, my goal is to illustrate the doable-ness of making simple changes and creating new habits one at a time to build a lifestyle of health even in the midst of busy mom life.

Drinking more water

I first started measuring my water intake during my third pregnancy. My first two babies had June birthdays, so between both pregnancies combined, I had the blessing of almost eighteen months of coolish weather. My third baby, though, grew throughout the second trimester right smack dab in the middle of summertime. Early on in the summer I noticed my hands were puffy. Worried that it was happening at only four months along instead of at the very end like it had with the other two babies, I mentioned the puffiness to my midwife. She suggested that I probably just needed to drink more water in the hot weather and should start measuring to make sure I was getting enough. *I drink tons of water,* I thought. *I'm always gulping out of a glass, and I pee constantly.* (Because peeing a lot is a really good measuring stick while pregnant, right?)

Using a thirty-two ounce Nalgene bottle, I started downing three full bottles per day. Lo and behold, it turns out that I hadn't been drinking even close to that before. It felt like a ton of water in the beginning, but being able to visually see the amount drain throughout the day made it so much easier, and I eventually got used to it. The puffiness in my hands disappeared quickly too! Now, years later, I still measure my water intake, and I love it! Because I'm not pregnant anymore, my intake goal has dropped to one and a half to two full bottles, but I still use the exact same system to track it. All you need is any water bottle or jug that has the ounces marked on it. Fill it up in the morning and you can easily track how much water you're actually consuming and set a goal for where you need to be.

Eating more fruits and vegetables

Eating more fruits and veggies can seem like a daunting task if you aren't used to it, but if this is one of your health goals for you and your family, some of these strategies may help. Many moms find that incorporating fruits and vegetables into already "accepted" foods helps make this nutrition goal much more achievable. Here are a few ideas (kids often like these options too, so bonus win):

Veggie Spaghetti Sauce—If you and your family are spaghetti fans, this suggestion can be a super easy way to hide extra vegetables in a meal. Whether you make your own sauce from scratch or just pop open a jar from the store (shout out to all my "spaghetti is what I make when I realize it's 4:30 p.m. and I haven't planned dinner yet" people), consider adding some thinly chopped or grated vegetables to the sauce and let it simmer long enough for the veggies to soften. I've added varying combinations of chopped spinach leaves, finely shredded carrots, bell peppers, onion, yellow squash, and zucchini. With all the seasoning and tomato goodness, the flavors tend to blend in quite well.

Fruit "Ice Cream"—If you have a blender, this recipe is an easy way to make a treat that's almost entirely fruit. Anything from chopped bananas to peaches or berries should work, as long as they're frozen. Fresh fruit can be sliced and thrown in a Ziplock bag to freeze, or you can find a lot of frozen fruit at the store. Just blend some of the frozen fruit on high until it's all ground up, then add a little milk (regular or nondairy both work) and stir them together until you have a smooth, ice-cream-like consistency. You can scoop it into a bowl or cone or heck, just eat it right out of the blender. It's good stuff!

Smoothies—Smoothies have become one of my favorite ways to get everyone in the family a blast of fruits and veggies, mostly because they're quick to make, everyone likes them, and all we need is a blender and some basic ingredients. We drink them regularly for breakfast or lunch as a convenient, healthy, go-to snack or even meal. I include things like raw spinach and carrots for a great, mild-tasting nutrition boost. There are lots of recipes out there.

Switching out snacks

Snacking can mean a range of things depending on whom you talk to, but if this is an area you're looking to change for the better, consider picking one or two healthy snack options to incorporate into your routine. Remember, building a healthier lifestyle usually isn't an all-at-once dive, it's finding what works for you and your family and changing things gradually until you have a routine you're satisfied with.

One of my normal routines with my husband now is having a cup of hot tea in the evening after we put the kids to bed. We'll sip it while we watch a movie, play Scrabble, talk, or listen to a podcast. It's become one of our "snacks."

Freshly popped popcorn (not the microwave stuff, but plain popcorn kernels popped either in an air popper or on the stove with a little olive or coconut oil) can be seasoned to taste (salt, garlic, basil, chili powder, or cinnamon and nutmeg for a sweeter route) and makes a light, super tasty snack.

Plain or lightly salted nuts, seeds, and almonds make an easy go-to snack, are nutritious, and are great mixed with dried fruit or a little bit of dark chocolate. If you've never tried a fresh apple, carrot, or banana spread with bites of nut butter, I highly recommend it!

Breaking a sugar habit

Several years ago my husband and I decided to go a whole month without excess sugar. Essentially, that meant no desserts and nothing sweetened (soft drinks, syrup on pancakes, sweetened yogurts, etc.). It was tough in the beginning, but we got used to it as the weeks went by, and it ended up being so worth it! Ever since then our bodies have less tolerance for sugar, we want it less, and sweet foods are not as appealing. A "sugar fast" like this may be a helpful step to take if eating less sugar is one of your health goals.

Again, these are just ideas, but I encourage you to identify one specific nutritional change you want to make, gather a strategy or two, and go for it. If the first strategy doesn't work, that's okay! Is there a way to step back and simplify it even more so it is sustainable? Maybe aim to have smoothies twice a week at first or maybe just skip added sugars one day a week. Perhaps focus only on drinking more water until that feels manageable, then build from there. As each small change becomes a norm, add a little more, and soon you'll find that the changes have turned into a whole new way of eating and drinking.

With a similar lens, let's take a look at fitness.

Fitness

Ah yes, fitness—a topic in the world of motherhood that can bring up anything from a sense of accomplishment and pride to guilt, frustration, and envy. We know we should exercise, and we know we want to look like we exercise, but for some reason, with many of us, it's like pulling teeth to actually get ourselves to create a real habit of exercising. Life gets in the way, kids need our time, we're tired, and working out gets pushed to the *someday* category.

I recently interviewed Rachel Aldrich Rader, a fitness coach who works specifically with moms. She explained that she teaches her clients to ask themselves, "Where can I move?" and then tells them to schedule it into their day or week. Some days this might be a solid block of time, and other days it might be little bits of time throughout.

Rachel's perspective helps so many moms because it takes away a lot of the I-should-be-doing-this-a-certain-way attitude that can often hinder us from making fitness progress. As a busy mom who wants to be healthier, your main key is to find something that works for you and your schedule. Find something that you can fit in your day, something that helps you move your body and work your muscles, and then start there. I'm personally not a gym person. I like using gyms, but it's just flat out not worth it to me to try and fit gym time into my week. I've found that I can be a lot more consistent by just planning home workouts and allowing myself to switch things up when I get bored with one certain type. I might make use of some workout videos for a month, then switch to jogs around the neighborhood with the kids in tow, then spend a while just doing various muscle exercises in the living room or backyard, then download a new workout app on my phone and use that until I want to do something else.

Some moms vastly prefer the gym setting and prioritize finding time to go so they can exercise without the kids, use the equipment there, or participate in certain workout classes.

Similar to nutritional goals, making a big fitness change all at once can be awfully hard to sustain. Starting small and building, however, can work extremely well. Remember, making lasting health changes takes time. If exercising at all seems completely overwhelming, believe me, I've been there, and so have many, many others! Consider setting one simple fitness goal that's doable for you and just start with that. Start with something you can maintain, schedule it in, and when you have the first step down, increase your goals. Again, we may not all have the same health goals, but this principle of piece-by-piece habit building can be extremely effective in the midst of a busy mom life.

Household

By *household health*, I'm referring to having a healthy living space. It can mean different things to different people, but the concept entails cleaning, decluttering, or whatever else is needed to keep our living environment healthy for ourselves and our families.

I admit that cleaning is not a high priority for me. I do enough to keep things decent, but that's about it. From personal experience and from speaking with other moms, I've learned that if you approach household health from the perspective of finding what works for you, it's much less overwhelming and far more likely to be consistent. This seems like an obvious statement, but here are a few examples:

I've never liked getting a bucket's worth of various supplies and lugging them to the bathrooms to clean everything. A couple of years ago someone introduced me to a super simple, inexpensive homemade cleaning spray, and ever since then cleaning the bathrooms feels way less tedious. Here it is, you ready? Fill an empty spray bottle with twenty-four ounces of water and one-third cup of white vinegar. Add approximately one teaspoon (more or less depending on preference) of your favorite scented essential oil or blend of oils (I love using peppermint!). Shake it up before using, and you're good to go.

Literally, this spray revolutionized cleaning for me. I use that one solution to clean basically everything, including mirrors. I know another mom who buys disinfectant wipes and cleans everything with those. Other moms do the bucket method and just keep a bucket of supplies under every sink in the house for easy access. There's no "right" way to do it, but whatever your preference, there's a way to keep things fairly quick and simple.

Let's take washing the dishes as another example. Good ol' never-ending dishes. To me, if the kitchen is clean, then the house as a whole feels clean. For years my husband and I would let the dishes pile up in the sink until the end of the day when one of us would finally tackle all of them. Some people prefer this method, but it always made everything feel messy to me. That was our habit though, and we kept it as the norm until we lived with my parents for three months during a move between cities. My parents, as empty nesters, never let dishes pile up. They empty the clean dishwasher in the morning, and after every meal, they immediately rinse and load the dirty dishes. After living there for a few months, my husband and I were both amazed to find how much we appreciated that method. We made a new habit of it while living there and have kept it as our way ever since.

Preferences and goals will differ in the realm of household health too, but if you can find some simple things that work for you and calm the overwhelm, it'll make a big difference!

I hope, precious Mothers, that this chapter has encouraged you in some way or another. All we physically and mentally go through daily as moms is no joke. Our health, for all its importance, can seem like a *back-burner* item or *hopefully someday* task in the chaos of raising children, running a household, and keeping up with other responsibilities. Whatever your health goals, I encourage you to view them as building blocks. Pick one or two pieces to start and go from there. Remember, you are you. You don't need to be anyone else. Find what works for *you*, and you'll be amazed at what you can accomplish. You've got this, precious Mama. You can do it. You can get there. **You are worth the process.**

Love your body
for what it is,
no matter it's
size, shape, or
the scars it may
bear.

~Melissa Smith
@love18smith

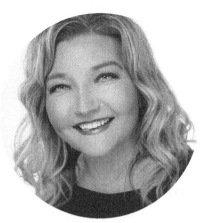

Melissa Smith

Melissa Smith is a best-selling co-author of the book, *You've Got This, Mama,* a health and wellness blogger, and an aspiring entrepreneur and teacher. She embraced 2018 as a year of growth and change both personally and professionally. She recently stepped away from a corporate management position to be a full-time mom and work toward her dream of spending more time with her husband and children through the pursuit of owning her own business and teaching.

Melissa aims to inspire others through her blog where she documents her own health and fitness journey after the birth of her third child. She has studied recreation and leisure, physical education, fitness, and strength training, and she is a certified teacher.

Melissa is creative, loves the outdoors, and has a passion for sun and surf. She enjoys meeting new people and building relationships. She is an eternal optimist and looks forward to experiencing new adventures awaiting in the future.

Ⓦ   healthymommy.ca

ⓕ   Younique Makeup by Melissa

ⓘ   @love18smith

~Special thanks to my incredible parents, Gordon and Helga Love, my amazing husband, Jeremy, and my fabulous children, Christopher, Benjamin, and Aliyah, for loving and supporting me unconditionally.

Five

GET HEALTHY, MAMA
Melissa Smith

"Nothing will work unless you do."
~Maya Angelou

It was October 2017 when I despised the reflection looking back at me in the mirror. I had just given birth to my third child a couple months earlier in August, and I knew I needed to do something about my body. I was pushing 220 pounds at that time, and I so desperately wanted to be a fit mama. I wanted to have the ability to run around and enjoy being active and playing with my children. I wanted to give my children a healthy mama who they could depend on—someone who would be present in their lives for as long as possible.

For as long as I can remember, I have struggled with my weight. When I was younger, it didn't seem to matter as much. I was always the chubby child (especially since my weight would fluctuate between my growth spurts) who would eventually sprout up and lose all the "baby fat." In high school I was very athletic, but I still found myself at the mercy of fat jokes and horrible nicknames. In my later school, college, and university days, I remained athletic and participated in sports and even worked at a local gym as a personal trainer. That time was a period in my life when managing my weight was possible without much effort since I was always busy engaging in physical activities. As an adult, those things became less important to me as I began focusing on my career and starting a family. Although I was a certified fitness trainer with an educational background in recreation and physical education with a focus on movement studies, I found myself in a fast-paced retail management career, which unfortunately meant eating at varying times of the day or night and often relying on quick and unhealthy food choices.

I began my weight loss and fitness journey in November 2017. There were no gimmicks, special programs or prepared meals, and no magic weight loss pills or protein shakes for replacement meals. It was a journey based on the simple foundation of caloric intake and output. Easy, right?! It certainly hasn't been the case for me. *Nothing worth having is ever easy, right?* I love food and I love to eat. I have always loved the idea of being fit too, but I would make excuses for myself—*I have no time to exercise or prepare meals, and my diabetes is a barrier.* In the past, my idea of healthy eating was not having a second helping of chips while watching TV or only having ice cream floats every other day. It was time for a change. I wanted to be a good role model for my kids and teach them how to properly nourish their bodies in a healthy way. I wanted them to know balance in their lifestyle choices.

My biggest hurdle is having type 1 diabetes and managing my disease with insulin pump therapy. Every time I exercised I needed to eat, and time after time I got discouraged because I never made any progress. In hindsight, I can see that this discouragement was always my biggest excuse. I decided that if I wanted to make a difference in my life, I needed to stop making excuses for all the reasons I *couldn't* do it and start focusing on the reasons I *needed* to. Having diabetes was not going to be my excuse any longer. In fact, it was even more reason for me to take care of my whole self. It wouldn't be easy, but I knew it was doable. I just needed to keep working at ways to make it work for me. I needed to be relentless.

I began by removing junk food from my diet and limiting the number of foods with refined carbohydrates or sugars in them. I focused on lean proteins, fruits, vegetables, and whole grains. I didn't totally restrict myself because I knew that would be more detrimental than good. Whenever I craved chocolate, I had a couple of pieces and savored them. If I wanted some cookies, I would have just one and relish every crunchy bite, but I mostly stuck to my healthy eating plan.

Over time it has become easier and easier to eat healthfully. I no longer crave those sugary and high-calorie, high-carbohydrate snacks. I enjoy shopping for new healthy foods, exploring new recipes, and spending time in the kitchen preparing meals. I share recipes with friends and family and have fun sharing photos and stories of my culinary experiences. I feed my family similarly but sometimes have a slight variation in what I make for myself, my husband, and my children. It is a whole family transformation. I initially worried that I would fail. I didn't want my transformation to be what my husband calls a "flash in the pan" where I decide I want to be healthy for a week and then fall off the wagon and back into my old eating habits. I refuse to call it a diet. A lot of people have asked me what it is I am doing. My answer? I am simply choosing to live a healthier, more active lifestyle—and it feels great.

When it comes to food, I often have to remind myself that although certain foods may taste great, they may not be the best choices for meeting my goals. I started researching the caloric needs for my age, gender, and level of activity, and the requirements for a postpartum nursing mom.

I did not want my desire to lose weight to interfere with the proper nourishment my baby needed. After determining the calorie range I required to lose weight, I spent a few days assessing how many calories I was consuming and then spent a few days observing *what* I was eating within that range. I haven't counted a calorie since. This journey is meant to be one that is flexible and attainable, and although much thought goes into making healthy choices, being too strict wouldn't work for me. In fact, being rigid in my approach would be detrimental, not sustainable, in the long run, and would send me running back to my old eating habits. The most important thing to do is to make decisions that work best for you to ensure your greatest success.

At the beginning of my wellness journey, I spent a lot of time looking at nutritional labels and recipes to get me started. My culinary skills have now evolved into experimenting with different flavors, spices, and food. I try to keep many healthy food options available in the house to choose simpler and healthier meals. I have become more creative in cooking meals that meet the needs and tastes of my husband and children as well. Some meals I make regularly include:

- Turkey meatballs with zucchini noodles and pasta sauce
- Lean ground turkey burgers served in lettuce wraps
- Baked pesto, tomato, and mozzarella chicken breast with spring mix salad
- Teriyaki chicken and zoodles (zucchini noodles)
- Deconstructed taco served on a bed of lettuce with salsa dressing
- Cauliflower crust pizza
- German beef rouladen with red cabbage
- BBQ chicken and vegetable kabobs
- Sesame bibimbap with riced cauliflower

Once I changed my eating habits and increased my water intake, I slowly added exercise and different activities to my schedule. I began walking to and from the kids' school and participating in aqua fit classes at my local recreation center twice a week. Since I am a mom of three, I have to be creative with my activities. I organize things that I can do with the kids like soccer in the backyard, basketball on the driveway, walks, bike rides, and dancing. At home, I add exercise into my daily activities including dancing while cooking, doing squat jumps while cleaning, running laundry up and down the stairs, and working out in the living room or the garage using the few pieces of equipment I have. There is *a lot* you can do without an expensive gym membership or any equipment at home. Be creative and innovative with your workouts—soup cans or juice jugs offer great resistance. Alternatively, you may prefer the variety or social aspects of what a gym, fitness center, or exercise program can offer. Do what works best for you and your family. The important thing is to be active consistently, however that fits into your lifestyle.

As my journey continued, my reasons for getting healthy also changed. I initially began my health journey with the intention of being thin and feeling comfortable with my reflection in the mirror. Now it is so much more than that—it's about being active and enjoying a longer life; it's about being strong and having endurance. As I continued to be consistent with my healthy lifestyle, I appreciated my body a lot more. Through all the aches and pains associated with working out and pushing myself, I began to really understand how important this body has been to me. It is the very vessel that carried and birthed my three beautiful babies. I now embrace my stretch marks because they are a reminder of what is so important in my life. The goal in this journey is not to be thin but to be healthy. Love your body for what it is, no matter the size, shape, or the scars it may bear.

I want to teach my children to have a healthy life too. I want them to live actively and to nourish themselves with food that will fuel their minds and bodies. This journey is about loving who I am—loving myself enough to take care of my body and accept no excuses. On your path to better health and wellness, you will certainly encounter obstacles. There will likely be things that stand in your way and people who will support you and people who won't. I call them "saboteurs." These are people who will tell you they feel you are doing something wrong, who send you unhealthy foods, or who encourage you to eat unhealthy foods. They will poke fun at you and scrutinize every detail about what you are doing. Try your best not to allow saboteurs to influence you and your decisions. Try not to let this behavior deter you in any way. Remember *why* you started your journey and keep those who truly support you close.

I have lost thirty-eight pounds since I began my journey. I still have more to go. After all, this is a marathon, not a sprint. There have also been many slip ups, setbacks, misfires, and restarts. Every time I wanted to give up I remembered how important it was for me not to forget why I started. For instance, I decided to enjoy the summer with my family and three children at home. Originally, I thought summer would be a great opportunity to kick things into high gear and have success. Instead, I found the time with my family so much more important. While I didn't completely give up on eating healthfully, I did enjoy the most special things in my life, which included ice cream treats. Once the kids were back at school, I was motivated to get back to having structure in the house again. I did not want to dwell on what could have been but to look forward to what is still to come. It was time to get my head back into it and refocus my energy. That I did, but from a different perspective. I needed to take care of other health concerns that became more important. I was suddenly hit with debilitating small fiber neuropathy that created a slight detour in my weight loss plans. I experienced the most painful burning skin sensation across the majority of my body, and the last thing I wanted to do was exercise. My mind was simply focused on the painful sensations I was experiencing during this time. I was taking medication that provided me with pain relief; however, doing so came with its own consequences and aftereffects of which weight gain was one. During this time of recovery, I also turned to my beloved food and gained back all thirty-eight pounds. I was pretty devastated, but I did not allow myself to sit in my tears for too long. I set out to do something important, and I was not going to let anything stop me. With the help and guidance of my neurologist and naturopath, I have since been able to wean off the medication I was taking and manage my new condition with the use of supplements, lifestyle changes, and nutrition. So here I am again, two years later, back at the starting line. However, this time I am not starting from scratch. I am starting from experience, and I know my rebuild will be stronger and more determined, yet gentler than before.

Health, I've learned, is something that should never be sacrificed—mentally, emotionally, or physically. While the initial goal to get fit and live a healthier lifestyle may stem from wanting to be a certain size or to fit into those pre-pregnancy clothes, consider making your long-term goal one of vibrant and renewed health. Go at your own pace but also challenge yourself while still listening to your body. If ever in doubt or unsure about something, seek the advice of a trusted professional and turn to your healthy mama community—be it in this book, in your local neighborhood, or online. If at some point you find yourself regressing into old patterns and behaviors, give yourself some grace, Mama. Be gentle with yourself. Listen to your body's cues. Whatever *being* healthy means to you, go do that. Start from a space of feeling good in your body, your skin, your soul, and your mind. Health will look different on every woman. Own your scars and stretch marks and be proud of your body, no matter what it looks like. You are enough. You created and carried life within you and birthed it. So give your body the caresses, gentleness, and love it deserves. Nourish it, nurture it, understand it, and above all, love it fiercely. Love yourself, Mama. **You've got this! You always have!**

I say, start now. Start where you are, but definitely start now.

- Tara Butterwick
@topknotmommy

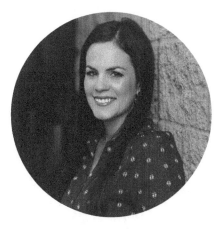

Tara Butterwick

Tara Butterwick has been told most of her life that she's mature beyond her years. We're not talking "old lady" mature. Instead, Tara is one to listen to others, bring laughter to their lives, and provide sound advice. She took a calling from an early age to help others. Her ability to find the joy in life is infectious. She is quoted by many as stating that *happiness is a choice,* and it's the mantra she has chosen to live by. Many regard her as ambitious with the thoughtfulness of always including others. She was born and raised in Calgary with strong moral values of love, connection, dedication, and support. It's no surprise that she has chosen to start and grow a business helping others while having two young children in tow. In fact, having children is what formed her business, drive, and mission.

Tara has always had a love for wellness. She left her corporate advertising career to pursue personal training, later branding herself *Top Knot Mommy* when creating a fitness business to help moms be fit, healthy, and real. She uses her position to grow community, lift up others, and spread positive fitness messaging in a world that so desperately needs it. She's been blazing a trail for thousands of moms and continues to unite, inspire, and motivate. As a dedicated voice in the fitness and wellness industry, Tara's future is bright. Funny, witty, passionate, and dedicated, she continues to do better for mamas and better for her community.

 topknotmommy.com

@topknotmommy

~ To my husband—who supports me to pursue my goals, pushes me to dream bigger, and constantly makes me laugh— thank you. To my two little babes: You changed my life in ways I can never put into words, and for this, I strive daily to show you just how much I love you. And lastly, to myself. You did it! The long nights after the kids are in bed, working to share your hustle and heart are so worth it. This is our story. And it made us stronger.

Six

THE POWER OF MOVEMENT
Tara Butterwick

*"Trade your expectation for appreciation and
your world changes instantly."*
– Tony Robbins

Let me start by saying that expectations are a natural part of life. However, they sure can lead to a mess that needs to be cleaned up when life happens and it's not how you imagined.

Let me also preface the above statement by saying I am an eternal optimist. I have always valued positive living and healthy lifestyle choices, but the quest for motherhood brought on challenges I didn't see coming and has led me to view healthy living from multiple perspectives. I believe you are in control of your own joy; nobody else has that power! Making healthy living a priority is a big part of that.

Now the truth is we all have expectations, but how do we deal with them? Expectations about conception, pregnancy, postpartum healing, what kind of mom we will be . . . the list goes on. But how do we move forward when they *don't* happen the way we dreamed? Can we use fitness positively and say *good-bye* to the concept of *losing baby weight* or *wearing pre-pregnancy clothes* to focus on our minds and nurture ourselves?

As a certified personal trainer, I have always taken good care of my body and my mind, and I have helped others do the same. It's my passion and what I truly love to do. When I became pregnant with my first at twenty-six years old, I was in the best shape of my life. I was fit, I had a tiny bump, and I felt amazing. I shake my head now for thinking those things mattered, and yet they don't at all. The thing is, I had never been pregnant before. I was one of the first of my friends to venture down that road. Every movie I had ever seen pertaining to pregnancy was all about crazy food cravings, loads of ice cream, really adorable maternity outfits, and chubby babies. You know, the picture-perfect life with the picket fence?

My expectation was to fit perfectly into that picket-fence bubble. After all, I am an optimist, so why wouldn't I? My story, however, was about to be rewritten. At thirty-one weeks and five days, I began getting Braxton Hicks contractions. But that's normal, right? Having felt a bit off for the entire morning, I called my doctor wanting reassurance that my cramps were simply Braxton Hicks. I went to the hospital to get checked. The good news was that there wasn't an infection. The bad news was that I was four centimeters dilated and fully effaced. This little baby was locked and loaded, and I was a sobbing mess. *But I am going out for dinner. The baby isn't coming for another two months. I am not ready for a baby yet. This is not part of my plan!* The sobbing continued and reality sank in. *My body was failing me, but worse, my body was failing my baby.* That's where my head went. I sat on bed rest for two days trying to keep the baby in. I felt so desperate to do right by my baby. When I couldn't hang on any longer, we welcomed a beautiful baby boy into the world. I barely saw him; he disappeared with a team of what seemed like ten neonatal intensive care unit specialists to get worked on immediately. All three pounds and fourteen ounces of him were part of me one minute and then gone the next. As I laid on my bed in a total blur, eating dry toast, I began to wonder what had just happened. I wasn't ready to be a mom, but in a way I was. He needed me, and in that moment, I needed to be needed.

Going home without my baby for weeks at a time while he was in the hospital forced me to question everything I knew about health, fitness, and what is truly important. I had just expected that my body could carry a baby full term. I honestly didn't know anything about the world of preemie babies. It changed my life. It changed me. It allowed me to see just how lucky we are. Our little boy is healthy, happy, and loved.

I soon learned that 8 percent of babies are born prematurely.[1] After learning this statistic, I wondered why. *Why me? Why my little boy?* When you have a preemie, doctors can't explain why a lot of the time. I didn't have an infection or any other condition, it was just my "little guy's time" or so I was told. I had to get out of the headspace that my body failed me. *But it did, right?* Or was that just the journey I was meant to have? I turned back to the best medicine I know—fitness—not to lose weight but to get my head straight. I rebranded my business to focus on mamas, and hence, **Top Knot Mommy** was born. I wanted mamas to feel empowered to be fit, healthy, positive, and real. Many mamas battle with something they didn't see coming; thus, a positive network and optimistic thinking are needed. These things helped me so many times. So I used fitness and teaching others to help heal my own wounds and to show myself how strong my body is, and I focused on using my story to help others so that they, too, could have this strong, tight-knit, open community.

When my husband and I looked into having another baby, the medical team let us know there was no reason why I couldn't carry full term.

They didn't have a reason for why I had had an early labor in the first place. It may or may not happen again, they said. I would be a high-risk patient, closely monitored by doctors, and I would take modified rest. Everything should be okay. Then, after a miscarriage, a meltdown, and a lot of questioning as to whether I was being greedy for wanting more children, we were very fortunate to get pregnant again. My dreams were coming true. My family was expanding. However, now I had a huge cloud of anxiety and fear I hadn't dealt with properly. I had a traumatic experience with my first and was thrown quickly into motherhood. I didn't really deal with the trauma. It was a dark cloud that came up like a crazy toddler tantrum. Around viability, I started to feel terrified that I wouldn't be able to keep this babe in. My baby needed me. *What if I couldn't do it?* But I had to. I remember telling my doctor, "Just hang me upside down if the time comes." Jokes are a coping mechanism for me, and I knew I might have to fight for this little baby.

With a chart the size of a dictionary (from all the visits, scares, and complications), I made it to thirty weeks. It was a huge win. It was all great until I started getting heaviness and the panic set in. Holy feck. It was happening again. I was dilated two to three centimeters and I needed to hold on with everything I had. In that moment, with a nineteen-month-old toddler at home, we decided I would go on full bed rest to keep baby in. Yet again, my mental fitness was being challenged, and I needed to pull myself together. I focused on self-care, on loving what I had, and on positive living. Making rainbows out of rainstorms is what you need to do sometimes to get through a tough situation.

Fast forward to Christmas. After being in and out of the hospital, I made it. I made it to thirty-six weeks. My relief was huge. I was *so* close. Two days later my water broke. This time I didn't cry tears of fear but tears of happiness. This was a big win for us—one I had hoped many long nights for. Lots of people I met at the hospital said, "Oh goodness! Only thirty-six weeks!" And here I was, happy beyond measure! That's the thing with perspective. Sometimes the things that happen to us in life provide a new depth of appreciation, a new lens to look through. Knowing what your mind and body are capable of is not always something we give ourselves gratitude for. Being mentally and physically fit and loving yourself *is* needed, and it's a recurring theme during postpartum.

Fast forward again through a groggy few months with **two kids under two**. I was back into fitness. I felt alive. Movement is therapy for my mind and my body, and I felt amazing. After being on rest and watching every movement while pregnant, I just wanted to use my body, move, and get that amazing stress release. I truly had never felt better. I was "superwoman." My expectation of having that part of my life back was coming together . . . that is until my crotch felt like it was going to fall out. That's right, it's all fun and games until your crotch is broken. I hadn't seen a pelvic physiotherapist between kids (which in looking back I should have), but I was pregnant three times in less than two years, so I didn't really know what was happening down there. This time I knew in my gut I needed to go get checked. Also, after having two kids and a high-risk pregnancy, where I was internally checked over and over, what's another set of fingers up there?

The next news shook me. I had a moderate prolapse. *Umm, what?* I legit pushed my adorable peanuts out and broke my insides. It's not like you can see anything, but your pelvic floor supports your internal organs and the heaviness is brutal. *I am a personal trainer. I am strong and in good shape. How does this happen?*

The real deal is that **it does happen**. The truth is, close to 50 percent of women will experience loss of pelvic organ support[2] regardless of which door your baby exited through: cesarean section or vaginal. It's. All. The.

Same! Many may be undiagnosed; many may just be living with symptoms. At the time, I didn't know a single person who had postpartum pelvic floor issues. I felt alone. I cried and questioned whether I would be able to chase my kids, exercise, or even do daily tasks without constant pain. *But why wasn't anyone talking about it? Surely, I am not the only one who is going through this.* The news devastated me.

I cried to my husband for about a week. I had lost myself in motherhood yet again. Yet I just felt like I had gotten "myself" back. *Was I being selfish? Is that just what we are supposed to give up? I love my babies, but who was I now? I felt like my body failed me. I couldn't keep a baby in full term, I broke my crotch, and yet I still had such an important role to do. I am their mom. And they don't care about those things.* They live in the moment, and I needed to do the same. I needed to get my head straight. I needed to let go of years of expectations and accept that these blips make me stronger. I needed to live for today and tomorrow, not yesterday—yesterday when I could run. I needed to get over that.

The huge list of exercises I couldn't do initially bummed me out. Then I put my big girl positive pants back on (it only took a week). I decided I needed to embrace what I **could** do. I needed to celebrate what my body did and love myself. I continued to go to pelvic floor physiotherapy, which is one of the first things I recommend to *anyone* postpartum. Go get checked out. Find out about your body and be your best advocate.

To get my shit together, I went back to my best form of therapy: fitness. This time I walked. I walked and I walked. I wasn't running like I used to, but I accepted that. I realized that power walking was safe for my body and gave me the mental clarity, stress release, and activity level I desperately needed. I focused on nourishing my body with healthy foods and using positive thoughts to change my perception. One of the most powerful things I did was talk about my journey.

I am a personal and group trainer.

I had two premature babies.

I have a moderate prolapse.

But that won't stop me. And better yet, it won't define me.

I am grateful for today and excited about the future.

The more I allowed myself to heal, the more it empowered me. It made my calling clearer. I spent years questioning, *Why me? Why my kids? Why my body?* Now I will make the best of my story to connect and share with others.

Movement is essential for life, and unfortunately, as mamas, we spend our days ensuring everyone else is taken care of and our wellness is left by the wayside. I say, start now. Start where you are, but definitely start now.

The role fitness and healthy living plays in our lives is completely woven into our mental health. It helps us see how strong our bodies can be and, in turn, creates a strength we can lean on. I believe it makes us stronger: stronger to take on the hard times and stronger to know what our minds are capable of. I now focus more on mental health and how exercise is crucial for a positive, happy mind.

No matter what kind of mama you are—stay at home, work at home, work out of the home—we all need movement. We all deserve to feel our best. After my journey, I have realized how much of our personal perceptions need a positive outlook; as mamas, we can't pour from an empty cup. Moving, nourishing our bodies, and positive thinking are essential for our lives and therefore must be a priority.

In the process of starting now, ask yourself: *Where is my fitness level?* If you haven't worked out since pregnancy or before, start slowly. Start where you are. If you have been working out, but not consistently, it's time to time block and make sure you know when you are working out and what you are doing. Remember, you aren't working out for before or after pics because your well-being isn't measured by that.

Don't listen to the media or the "how to lose five pounds in six minutes" garbage. It's not real. You are real; your heart is real. So move because it fills up your soul, it brings you sanity, and because it just feels so dang good.

Here are my top tips to set you up for success, to get your head in the game, and to make yourself a priority:

When are you working out? In the morning? Nap time? Can you put on a twenty- to thirty-minute show and get a workout in? Can you get out walking daily? Do you have access to a gym that has childcare? Are you more energetic at night? *Whatever* your jam, decide your **when** and be disciplined with your time. Honor that commitment.

What will you do? Now that you have a time block, you need to know exactly what you are doing. Are you doing a twenty-five-minute workout at home? Are you going to power walk followed by squats? Are you hitting that class at the gym when your partner gets home from work? Figure out the **what** so you have a solid plan.

Now this may seem like a shock, but number three is the one I hear time and time again as being the hardest. **You need to do it**. You need to make it happen. You know when and what, so you have to use your mental strength to get it done.

Okay, so you're ready. You are excited to get into a routine. Start today. Whether it's five minutes, ten minutes, or an hour. Start today. Then commit to three times a week. Do that for three weeks, and then keep going.

Need inspiration for what your workouts could look like?

- Power walk with your tribe for thirty to forty-five minutes, three times a week

- 7:00 a.m. workouts Monday, Wednesday, and Friday while the kids play/watch a show. Twenty-five minutes of strength, cardio bodyweight exercises
- Two power-thirty walks every week with squats, lunges, and modified push-ups at the end *with* one kid-free workout at your favorite fitness studio

Heck, sometimes it's ten minutes of strength exercises in the morning, chasing kids *all day*, and then ten minutes of squats and squat pulses while cooking dinner. *But* getting into movement will get you out of your funk. You see, it's the consistency of movement, of finding what works for you!

Want to get more educated, but aren't sure where to look? Here are some amazing in-the-know resources for postpartum fitness information/ programs:

- Jessie Mundell's 8-week Core + Floor Restore
- Mutu System Program
- Moms Gone Strong

Once you get started, a beautiful thing will happen. Your mindset will get stronger, and you will feel like you can tackle *anything* your day or life brings you. I personally need fitness now more than ever, more than any of the hard times before. I am thankful that I was able to use the power of movement to heal, adjust, adapt, and grow. Do it for you. Do it to be the *best* version of yourself to share with your family.

You see, I expected I would have three kids. *Here we are, back to expectations.* I didn't see the journey we had coming. Nobody does. But I can work on the now to be my best self. I can navigate the waters of assessing the risk of premature labor. *Is another child right for our family? Could we even get pregnant?*

Nobody is perfect. Grace is required. But you need to know that only *you* can control your daily happiness. You see, fitness is one thing that *only you* can do for you. You have to earn it. You can't buy it. So together let's shake off modern weight loss, post-baby body BS, and get moving. Let's start loving ourselves and *everything* we have achieved. It's time to say *see ya* to expectations, to make ourselves a priority, and to be mentally and physically fit for anything life sends our way! **#youvegotthis**

When I slow down, it creates a sense of spaciousness for life to unfold the way it should.

~Hillary Dinning
@drhillarynd

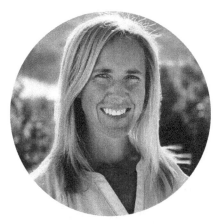

Hillary Dinning

Hillary Dinning is a naturopathic doctor based in Calgary, Alberta. Her practice focuses on fertility, postpartum, prenatal, pediatrics, and chronic conditions. A graduate from the University of Western Ontario with an undergraduate degree in kinesiology, Hillary knew she wanted to pursue a career in naturopathic medicine. After spending eight years in a finance role, she was ready to switch gears. In 2010, Hillary commenced her doctoral degree in naturopathic medicine at the Canadian College of Naturopathic Medicine. Going to work now feels like going home—this is what she is meant to be doing. As much love as she has for her work, however, her heart belongs to her family. Her children, Barrett (Bear), Tucker, and Isla, along with her husband, Dave (Smitty), provide endless amounts of love, laughter, light, craziness, and mayhem in her life. A perfect day in the life of Hillary Dinning would include morning cuddles with her family, time outdoors, a long mountain trail run, a warm Epsom salt bath, a good dose of laughter, a delicious glass of wine, and a plate of freshly baked chocolate chip oatmeal cookies. Connecting with people fills Hillary to the brim. She loves life and lives it wholeheartedly.

 doctorhillarynd.com

Dr.Hillary

@drhillarynd

~I dedicate this piece to my life teachers, Barrett, Tucker, and Isla: Your unguarded hearts, ears, and eyes encourage the best Me to show up every day. To my love, Smitty: You have gifted me space to grow and provide humor at the best possible moments. And to my sister Alex for showing me what unconditional love is.

Seven

LETTING GO
Hillary Dinning

"In the end these things matter most: How well did you love? How fully did you live? How deeply did you let go?"

~Jack Kornfield

Control Freak

I have most people fooled. I seem pretty laid back when it comes to life; however, the laid-back attitude can only show up when I have things *all under control.* And most of the time I do. Right now, though, I'm hanging on by a thread. Life is busy—busy with three little beings to help grow and nurture, to drive to lessons, school, and playdates, all the while still finding quality time to connect with a husband who is running just as fast as I am toward life, career, and everything in between. My life is busy with a career I'm in love with and could spend hours learning new information about. Additionally, with running a household and investing time in myself, like I said, I'm hanging on by a thread.

My controlling nature has shown up differently throughout my life. Growing up, my nightly routine involved arranging my pillows and covers over my head in a very specific way before I even dreamed about relaxing into sleep. The sense of security that I had when these physical objects were around me in *just* the right way allowed me to feel like *I* was in control, not the boogeyman who might approach me. In my teenage years and well into university, my tight grip on life showed up in the friends I chose. I made sure I had just the right, tight, close-knit group of friends around me—so I could control how I felt, so my comfort zone was set. In my early career years, I took a path that didn't fully resonate with who I ultimately am, so control took on the form of drive; I was driven to prove my worth and earn the title of "successful" in something that did not come naturally to me. When I stepped into my second career as a naturopath, and then started having babies, control morphed into being busy. I like to jam in as much as I possibly can in a given day. I feel like I'm in a perpetual, seemingly never-ending race most of the time: a race to ensure everyone and everything around me is taken care of; a race to check things off my list. The cortisol surge that comes with *checking things off my list* is addicting. Ridiculous, right? I know! Furthermore, staying still is actually very uncomfortable for me. It makes me feel vulnerable and alone, and therefore insecure and sad. The more I strive to control everything around me, the more I feel like I'm *doing*, and the more I accomplish things, the more I feel safe and secure.

The very real possibility that this isn't the truth—that having so much control is, in fact, not the healthiest thing for me, either physically or emotionally—has been knocking at my door for quite some time now. There were times in the past when I opened the peephole to speak to it, but I never welcomed it or embraced it—the door would be slightly open, not too wide, not too tight, just enough to say, *Hi, hello, I see you, but I need to continue the way I've been going on because that is all I have ever known.* Only over the last few years have I invited this truth to come in and stay a while. It would be nice to say that the ending to this story is *we lived happily ever after*. That's just not the case, though. Truly, we are right in the juiciest part—the part when the dance-off takes place between me and this lesson of letting go.

Opening the Peephole

All three of my children have played a significant part in teaching me to let go of control and trust that life will work out the way it's supposed to. It always does. *Trust* is the key word here.

I am learning to trust that I am supported, I am guided, I am always taken care of by the Universe when I let her show up for me—she truly does have my back. This is a tough one to put into action because it requires me to leave behind the ever-spinning wheel of medical knowledge, over-thinking, over-analyzing, and to be more centered and present in my body. I believe this is where our intuition—that *gut instinct*—and our real *knowing* lies, as opposed to the mind racing in our brain. I'm realizing that when I can act according to what this voice tells me, I resonate more with the Universe and her grand plans for me. I can loosen that white-knuckle grip on my life, the one I have held so tightly since childhood, and *let go. Breathing in spaciousness. Trust. Breathe. Repeat.*

My Birth Journeys

None of my birthing journeys went the way I planned or envisioned. Not even one thing came close to the strategically mapped picture in my head. However, looking back on each of them, there were magical moments. No stars and swooning music—just exact moments when, right in the center of my gut, deep down in my "knowing," I knew that

I was exactly where I was meant to be, feeling exactly what I was meant to feel, and walking the exact path I was meant to walk.

Like Old Friends

With my first pregnancy, I assumed I would have a natural delivery. Smitty and I even decided we'd have our child at home. I was popping natural birth-prep remedies, sticking capsules of cervix softeners up my wahoo, and taking all the right supplements, so I naturally thought, "I've got this!" Although I was quite set on having a home birth, I was very open to all possibilities—all except one: a cesarean section.

At forty-two weeks, I was a bit discouraged when my water only partially broke on the ultrasound table and my midwives told me to head to the hospital. I knew in my gut I wasn't going home that day. It was one intervention after another. The medical staff fully broke my water, put me on Pitocin (to induce labor) and then kept hiking up the dose with each hour that passed.

I remember when the fear crept in like shadows in the crevices on a dimly lit cobblestone alley. I remember when I left my breath and body and shifted back into my head like a mouse on a wheel. Fear is a powerful emotion. It overtakes your gut instinct. Shortly after the fear crept in, and fifty-two hours of labor later, I chose the option of speeding up the process and delivering via cesarean section.

I was promptly wheeled into the surgical room. Instead of finding a bright, sterile room like we see in the movies, I was welcomed by what sounded like a group of buddies sharing stories over pints at a local pub. It felt like a warm welcoming. The surgeon was from my hometown, and the anesthesiologist was from Smitty's hometown, and we proceeded to join the table and get in on the story sharing. The ease in which Barrett came into this group of people, the happy cries from my husband when he held his firstborn, my joy in hearing it was a boy, the look on Barrett's face as he was handed to me over the curtain—I will never forget. Herein lies the magical moment.

I didn't struggle with my decision to deliver Barrett via cesarean. Where I struggled was how I started equating my inability to let go of control and trust the process with my inability to have a vaginal birth. Over the next four years, I started to figure out how to navigate this intimidating/enlightening journey of "letting go."

Warmth in and amongst the Sterility

With my second pregnancy, I was determined to do it right with the goal in mind of having a natural birth. With the intention of opening up my pelvic area, I switched from running to more yin exercises such as yoga. I started meditating, working with my breath, and learning visualization techniques to create a welcoming and open environment through my vaginal canal. Running had been my escape, so letting go of it and doing these other activities was a big deal to me. It felt like a sacrifice, one that, in my view, would ensure that this delivery would unfold the "right" way.

I felt really good toward the end of my pregnancy—I was in a good head space, and more importantly, I felt like I was finally *out of my head and present in my body.* By forty-one weeks and three days, my body still had not progressed. No effacement, no dilation, nada. Zip, zilch.

I remember the moment when I was no longer present in my body, when all that energy transmuted to mind energy instead. It was the afternoon of forty-one weeks and three days when, according to "medical guidelines," I should be getting induced. Knowing what occurred after my last induction and knowing that I was not even close to being dilated or effaced, I decided that induction was not the way I wanted to go. I was given the choice to either wait until forty-two weeks (which was in four days) or go the following morning at 6:00 for a cesarean section! Smitty and I discussed our options, but I was adamant I would deliver my baby the following day. I felt headstrong, hot and bothered, and ready to roll. Then I realized that these feelings could be related to my inability to stay out of my head and in my breath and body. Perhaps in the next four days things would change? Perhaps I needed to give my body more time to go where it was supposed to? And so the battle raged between my head and my gut. In the end, I thought of a thousand reasons why we should go in for a cesarean the next day. And so we did.

The cesarean section for my second child, Tucker, went a lot differently. This time it felt sterile and devoid of any humor, any emotion. It was eerily cold and very procedural—it felt like I was in the wrong place at the wrong time, that is until Smitty announced I had birthed a boy rather than the baby girl I was certain I was carrying. I remember feeling the room fill with love, feeling the sterility change to warmth. I cried this time as my heart broke open to this little gem. *You've surprised me, my sweet boy, and somehow I know that this is the first of many times that your little soul will do just that.* Herein lies the magical moment.

After Tucker's birth, having done everything "right" to prepare myself for a vaginal birth, the realization that there's more to the birth path than what I was "doing right" dawned on me. And so I slowly opened myself to the idea of surrendering control, surrendering the tightly held blueprint of the dos and don'ts during pregnancy and life's journey thereafter, surrendering myself to the idea that there is something bigger than I am, and knowing that I am supported every step of the way.

A Fairy Visit

During my third pregnancy, I went the completely opposite way. I did absolutely nothing to prep—no vaginal cervix softeners, no *delicious* herbal tinctures, no homeopathic remedies, and definitely no meditating. Nothing. I didn't put a lot of thought into my delivery. I also didn't switch to being present in my body. I ran around like a bat out of hell, between working my job and running after my two small "looney tunes"!

Having had two cesareans under my belt, my midwives had me schedule yet another cesarean section. However, they agreed to book it at the latest possible date they were comfortable with: forty-one weeks and three days. Five days prior to my actual due date, I felt the contractions. These surpassed what I thought Braxton Hicks contractions felt like; they were the "stop mid-step and breathe through this" type of contractions. You can imagine my excitement! They would come on strong, crescendo, and then quiet down at certain points of the day and night. At each crescendo I was certain that this was the time; this was the time that this babe was coming out my vagina!

My body worked hard up until the morning of forty-one weeks and three days. That morning, oddly enough, contractions stopped almost completely. While I sat in the waiting room to head to my cesarean for Isla's birth, an obstetrician who had been following my case a week earlier for other reasons came by to introduce herself. She ended up being a fairy godmother in disguise! She said, "I know your intention was to have a vaginal birth, and I'm sorry that didn't work out for you." She went on to explain that she is very pro-vaginal birth after cesarean (VBAC), even after two of them, and that my situation just *is* what it *is*. I told her I had been experiencing pre-labor pains for five days, and she asked if I was interested in having her examine me to see how far I had progressed and was dilated, if at all. Even though it turned out I wasn't progressing, *this* was the final piece of the puzzle that allowed me to understand completely that the cesarean section that was about to take place was meant to be. Herein lies the magical moment.

Hindsight

In hindsight, all my births were meant to go the way they did. Instead of feeling put to the test to let go of control, I realize now that they *went the way they went*; they were beautiful events surrounded by immense love and magic. This realization has played a major role in allowing me to actually *let go*.

Life with Children: The Lesson Continues

Birthing Barrett, Tucker, and Isla was just the beginning. Hanging out with these tiny humans—guiding them, nurturing them, loving them, laughing with them, and crying with them—is a whole other ball game. I keep us all busy with activities—teaching them, stimulating them, and relaxing them. It's a lot of *doing* still. It is only more recently that I started to understand the concept of *slowing down to speed up*.

Slow Down to Speed Up
Slowing Down

To me, slowing down means having the ability to walk through life while being present in every moment and experiencing it to the fullest instead of rushing and running all the time and constantly chasing one thing after the other. It means loosening that white-knuckle grip.

I put slowing down into practice in different ways, like letting our days unfold on the weekends instead of having a set schedule. Additionally, something as simple yet profound for me is staying behind a car going the speed limit instead of darting around it or switching lanes to get ahead. Slowing down also shows up in my relationship with my husband—allowing a conversation or argument to play out over time instead of being *solution based* within that one time and space. I am placing more intention on allowing what is to *just be*. I'm learning to recognize the difference between getting cross with our children for bad behavior versus snapping at them because I'm feeling a loss of grounding and control in other aspects of my life. Now, *sometimes* I can back away and catch my breath before my interactions with them spin out of control. In my naturopathic medicine practice, slowing down looks like quieting my medical brain and allowing my intuition to guide part of my decision making as I build patients' treatment plans.

> *"I have actually considered that love just might be the opposite of control." ~Glennon Doyle*

Speeding Up

When I slow down, it creates a sense of spaciousness for life to unfold the way it should. It can show up as a perfectly cozy and lazy Saturday morning, followed by a fun outing with the five of us. It can show up as a successful treatment plan for a patient or a harmonious relationship with my husband. It can be as simple as staying behind a slow-moving vehicle and actually beating the cars in the fast lane! And it can be something as big and bold and beautiful as watching my children grow into their very own individual personalities.

Trusting That I Will Show Up: Recovering after a Cesarean Section

Sher Doward, a teacher and mentor of mine once shared this thought with me: Trusting that the Universe has your back allows you to spend less negative or forceful energy keeping everything in line *and* to know that if anything were to go off the rails, *you* are the exact person who will show up for *you*. *You* will know how to help yourself or others. *You* will be able to manage a situation and rise to the occasion. Trust this inner *knowing* to be true, trust *you* . . . explicitly. This is exactly what happened when I was recovering from my cesareans.

I don't remember exactly how I came up with my recovery protocol. Was it pulled from my fresh-out-of-school brain? Did it intuitively just *feel right?* I imagine it was a mixture of both. What I do know is that it has served me differently in its special way after each birth.

My formula includes the following:

Homeopathic remedies. Used for bruising, emotional trauma, inflammation, pelvic tissue trauma, and nerve pain. I popped these little guys like candy from day one. These are my painkillers and physical healers.

Scar healing. I once read an excerpt in *Chicken Soup for the Mother's Soul* that referenced what a mother wanted to tell her daughter who was deciding to have kids: "I want her to know that a cesarean scar or shiny stretch marks will become badges of honor."[2] And that's just what they are. With my first cesarean, I couldn't touch my scar without feeling a little scared of it—it felt ropey and was quite sensitive. What I've realized, though, is that through exploring the scar tissue with my fingers, rubbing calendula oil and vitamin E on it, and allowing my hands to comfort it, it has slowly become a part of me, a part of my story.

Stability exercises. All my abdominal muscles became a bit disheveled and stretched during pregnancy and were torn, especially during my last cesarean. I worked with a Pilates instructor who showed me a daily routine of stability exercises I could do to heal my abdominal wall and get my running muscles back! Over time, though, I realized that it was becoming too much about the routine and less about listening to what my body needed, so I started listening and then transformed these exercises.

Osteopathy work. I often explain to patients that osteopaths take the same holistic approach to healing as naturopaths; however, osteopaths do gentle physical work on the body. This work helps to mobilize and support the body in its re-shifting of muscles, bones, and organs back to *normal* postpartum.

Time. Spending time in bed, in my house, and hanging out with babe. *This is an obvious one, right?* For me, time became the most important factor after my three births. With Bear's birth, I couldn't wait to get out of the house. I even bundled him up in a blanket the day I got home from the hospital and walked to the end of my block and back. I laugh thinking about it—my ab muscles were nonexistent, and my boots were so heavy they hurt my back. With Isla, I promised myself seven days without leaving the house. On the fifth day, I went outside in the backyard, and even though I didn't quite make it to seven, I really valued this time.

And So the Dance Goes On

Loosening my grip on life is a lesson in progress. I'm constantly learning to shift and evolve from how I am naturally programmed—consciously choosing to break patterns that have been around for almost forty years (*that's a long time, heh?!*). I'm growing as a woman in business, as a mother to my children, as a wife to my husband, and as a friend and a source of strength and support to myself. My children, each in their own way, have provided me with this opportunity. I will be forever grateful. And so the dance goes on. That "get yer funk on, wiggle your behind, shake your wrists, point your fingers to the sky, sing along, wild and crazy" type of dance.

Section 2

MIND

Featuring
Amanda Archibald

Tania Jane Moraes-Vaz

Mona Sharma

Andrea Taylor

Christina Whelan Chabot

Jodi Decle

OPENING COMMENTARY BY
Sabrina Greer

When you hear the word *mind*, what do you think of? Do you picture your actual brain and the functions of each area? Is it pink and resemblant of an enormous blob of chewed bubble gum? Do you think about artificial intelligence (AI)? Maybe a good sci-fi movie? Or do you think of something deeper, like consciousness, the unseen? You are using your mind right now to read this book and answer these questions. The **mind** is comprised of all your cognitive faculties including *consciousness, perception, thinking, judgment, language,* and *memory.*[1] The mind is potentially the most important element of our health; it is what tells us *how* to perceive our feelings and how to process and communicate our thoughts. It is our mind that sends the message to our pain receptors and triggers a physical response in our body. This is the mind-body connection. You have likely felt "butterflies" in your tummy when you are nervous. Mind-body connection. When discussing health and the mind, if we use the guide of soundness and the holistic approach (meaning *being whole*), we can view the body, mind, and spirit as one.

In this section, we dive into a mother's psyche and speak to all the challenges and astronomical life changes that motherhood brings. Did you know that one in seven mothers experiences postpartum depression (PPD)?[2] Postpartum depression awareness is growing, but often this debilitating condition goes undiagnosed due to the ugly stigmas and judgments connected to the word. As mamas, we feel such shame attached to any emotion other than joy. *This is supposed to be the best time of my life, right? I should be grateful, I mean, I am grateful. What's wrong with me? I am a horrible mother, woman, person. Who thinks this way? I don't deserve to be a mama.* Sound familiar? I am pretty sure we have all been there, PPD or not, diagnosed or not. It is completely normal to have feelings of inadequacy and self-doubt. Even for us teachers with degrees in developmental psychology and three children, we still have days where we question our abilities.

It is normal to feel new stresses and anxieties when you suddenly have new responsibilities and an abundance of unknowns. Postpartum depression can actually last for years and has a spectrum, making it difficult to recognize. I remember the emotions I personally experienced in early motherhood were loneliness, resentment, fear, and guilt. **Loneliness** because of the absence of adult conversations and nights out with my girl gang. **Resentment** because the majority of the household workload fell on *my* already bruised lap while my husband *got* to go out to work. **Fear** for pretty much everything, but mostly for keeping this tiny human alive. Oh, and the **guilt**. I felt such deep guilt for everything: how I was feeling, what I was thinking, the things I was doing and not doing. It was (and often still is) exhausting.

I love my kids more than anything in the world, just like you do yours, but each age and season brings with them new challenges and roller coasters of emotions. In trying to become a mama, there can be so much anxiety and stress that accompanies the process. *Once you see those double lines, it becomes worth it, doesn't it?* When you are a new mama, there are the obvious obstacles: physical and emotional adjustments, lack of sleep, and changes in relationships and life as you previously knew it. *Those delicious baby snuggles make it all worth it though, don't they?* Then, of course, there are toddler tantrums and picky eating and independence and potty training . . . did I say tantrums already? *Watching the synapses fire in those tiny brains as they learn and master new skills is worth it though, isn't it?* What about making lunches, mood swings, parent/teacher meetings, sports, school trips, and permission slips? And don't even get me started on homework. *Watching them express their individuality and personality is worth it too though, right?* How about that teenage angst? That everything-is-the-end-of-the-world attitude. Real relationships and friendships. Social media. Borrowing (or in some cases stealing) the freaking family car? *Knowing you did the best you can to raise a kind human being is why we sign up for this journey in the first place though, I am sure of that.*

Please know, Mama, that we are not here to judge. Motherhood is HARD with a capital H.A.R. and D. There is really no way to prepare. There are no books, guides, or instruction manuals on how to manage motherhood, only sharing our truths to affirm that we are not alone in this journey. This section candy coats nothing. We dive into all the difficult and raw emotions associated with every stage of mental motherhood. It never gets easier, it is fluid and ever changing, it ebbs and flows. Every stage is a season, some stormier than others, some dry, and some unpredictable. When it comes to health and the mind, it is important to remember that just like the body, we must nourish her, be gentle, kind, and loving with her. We must not judge our mind harshly or set unrealistic expectations. The brave warriors in this section bare all. They share their intimate journeys and speak up about mental health to provide hope. There will be tough days and hurricanes, but there will also be so much joy and the sunniest of skies. Please just always remember that wherever you are in your story, **you've got this, Mama.**

You are the one who can give your children a happy mother, and that's all that matters.

~Amanda Archibald
@amandathemamacoachvan

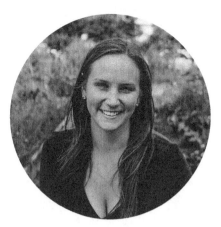

Amanda Archibald

Amanda has always been known for her caring and empathetic nature. Her positive outlook in life has been her strong suit as she navigated school and nursing and while running her own business and journeying through motherhood. She is a mom to one little girl, is the wife to an amazing husband, and she lives in Vancouver, BC, Canada.

Amanda received her Bachelor of Science in Nursing, with a specialty in perinatal nursing, from the British Columbia Institute of Technology. She worked in labor and delivery as well as postpartum care in Vancouver and Calgary before having her own daughter. Shortly after her daughter's birth, Amanda struggled with the overwhelming amount of information new mothers receive. Her baby had a challenging temperament, and she felt alone in her journey. She wished for more guidance and support. Inspired by this desire, she launched her business, *The Mama Coach - Amanda Archibald*, in Vancouver, a coaching and support service for new mothers. She is an International Board Certified Lactation Consultant (IBCLC), an infant and child sleep consultant, and a prenatal educator who provides support and guidance to new mothers! Her mission is to help make motherhood easier by building community through education and connection.

🅦 themamacoach.ca/Amanda-Archibald

📷 @amandathemamacoachvan

~ To the girl who made me a mother, who thrives in my failures and grows in my strengths. My Emily, my best friend, my partner in this journey of motherhood. Thank you for being the mirror in my life that shows me where I need to grow, and for pointing out all the obvious things I hide from. I hope you never lose your spirit, my little girl.

Eight

SHARING MY TRUTHS SO SHAME CANNOT SURVIVE
Amanda Archibald

"If we can share our story with someone who responds with empathy and understanding, shame cannot survive."

– Brené Brown

I knew something was wrong. I had an uneasy feeling from the moment I found out I was pregnant. This feeling is the downside to pregnancy after miscarriage. Having just lost my first baby a month prior, I was flooded with emotions including fear and anxiety of the unknown. I had about two seconds of joy before the real feelings set in. *What if I lose this baby too? How am I supposed to feel happy with another potential for loss?* I went straight into my nursing role and medical mind: I wanted every ultrasound and all the blood tests done before I could feel the *realness* of this pregnancy. Working for five years as an obstetrical RN had skewed my view of pregnancy. When you are on the front lines experiencing all the complications pregnancy has to offer, it is hard to believe your pregnancy can be normal. When I told friends about my insecurities, everyone tried to reassure me, but my mommy instincts told me I would lose my second baby too.

It was a cold Sunday afternoon when I bled. We headed to the hospital, and I knew we would come home with another loss in our hearts. It is a surreal feeling to be on the receiving end of this news. I sat on the triage bed where I had seen patients just days earlier. But this time *I* was the patient and this loss was *mine*. For weeks following this loss, I became obsessed with trying to determine why: *Why did this happen to me? What did I do wrong? Why had my body failed me?* All I ever wanted was to become a mother, and I was failing. When you get pregnant, you imagine that you will get to meet your baby, and you start imagining your life with children. I was making plans, and when I miscarried, I didn't just lose my babies, I lost my future as well.

Instead of grieving my losses or dealing with the emotions, I threw myself into research. *How could I prevent this from happening again? How could I get pregnant again?* I purchased ovulation tests and pregnancy tests and scheduled and planned around the clock. It was all I could think of. I'd spend hours scrolling through social media and reading stories similar to mine. I did this for hope, but also for research. *How did they get pregnant again? Did they change their diet, did they use any particular supplement(s), or did they see a fertility doctor? How could I be the best at conceiving a child without failing again?*

The planning and research worked because I found myself pregnant just four short weeks later. When I took a pregnancy test, I feigned excitement. My heart pounded, partly from excitement, but mostly out of fear. I was so focused on becoming pregnant that I didn't really think about how to handle myself and the emotions that would come after. I walked out of the bathroom and saw my husband sitting on the couch. I uttered the words, "Well, we are pregnant again . . ." As we hugged each other, I could feel the tension rise between us. The air felt thick and heavy like I could slice it with a knife. I could tell right away we felt conflicted with our emotions. We were happy about this pregnancy, but our past losses overshadowed a moment that should have felt like absolute bliss. I felt numb and disconnected—from myself, my body, and this baby, all a façade of self-preservation. As I climbed into my bed that night, I put my hands on my belly and prayed to whoever might listen, the same way I did as a child whenever I wished for a sunny day so I could play outside: *Please keep this child, please let me meet her, you are my greatest joy and my biggest fear.* This moment is when my obsessive behavior escalated. I took twenty-five pregnancy tests over the next week, hoping to see a darker and darker line. I went to the bathroom every hour just to wipe and ensure I wasn't bleeding. As soon as we could detect a heartbeat, I would wake in the night to use a Doppler.

We waited until I was twenty weeks pregnant before sharing our news, and even then I remember feeling some hesitation. *Should we do this?* Sharing the news of our pregnancy made it feel more real, and I think part of me still felt more comfortable that we'd kept it under wraps. If we told people we were expecting a baby, they would be excited, and I would have to feel excited too. I would have to feel something for this child, which made the potential loss so much greater to bear. In order to never feel the same pain again, I was doing everything I could to emotionally distance myself, completely disconnect from feeling anything for this baby. No feelings, no pain.

I spent nine months growing this beautiful human, all while harboring these feelings, tensions, and stressors. Although I truly wanted to connect with this baby, it seemed impossible at the time. I felt like she was a separate entity. My anxiety had crippled me and debilitated me by disconnecting me from both the situation and my life. I struggled to be a good wife, daughter, sister, and friend. I couldn't feel the joy that everyone was expecting from me, so I removed myself. As I approached my due date, I doubted my abilities as a mother. *How could I not bond with this baby I had so badly wanted? What kind of terrible person would feel so numb about bringing new life into this world?*

Emily was born surrounded by loving and caring souls. I remember the nurse saying it was a "perfect delivery." I couldn't have agreed more; it was textbook. My labor was normal, there were no complications, and a beautiful baby was born and placed onto my chest. She was real, this was all very real, and for the first time ever I felt the weight of motherhood.

We were discharged from the hospital the next day. We packed up our teeny, tiny babe and made our way home on a cold November day. We got home and placed her car seat on the floor in the living room so our dog could sniff her. I sat on the couch and thought, *Now what?!* You see, throughout the last nine months, I was mainly focused on delivering a healthy baby into this world, and now here I was, in my house with my baby, and I had absolutely no idea what to do with it . . . with her. I wanted to bond with her, to feel that instant connection of love that everyone talks about, but I truly didn't have that; she felt like a stranger to me. I had spent a lot of time preparing for her—baby gear, clothes, cooking, cleaning, and nesting . . . but I had spent no time preparing *myself* for her.

On our first night at home, my husband took the night *shift* so I could rest, and when it was my turn to be up, I felt this strike of anxiety hit me like a ton of bricks. He went to bed, and I sat crying (*which I did a lot of postpartum*) in the living room, staring at her in her baby swing. She stirred, so I picked her up, assuming she was hungry. I propped up all my pillows so I could breastfeed her with ease. She latched on, my milk came in rather quickly, and I thought to myself, *Wow, this could be our*

thing . . . I could be good at this . . . I could master this . . . I can feed you.
I then became obsessed with breastfeeding.

You see, I calm my anxieties with obsessions; it is something I have done my whole life. Whenever life feels overwhelming or uncertain, I move to things I can control, often gaining knowledge on the topic as the first step. In this case, I learned everything I could about breastfeeding. I knew some things before I had a baby, but now it was a whole new game. I also became a little possessive of my girl. I felt like I had missed out on so many months of getting to "know" her while she was in utero that I had to make up for lost time. Every chance I could get, I took her into a quiet room and nursed her, away from visitors or chaos because I wanted *my* time: mommy-and-Emily time. Even when I felt frustrated or exhausted on all fronts, I couldn't bring myself to leave her. I wanted . . . I *needed* to spend every moment making up for the mistake I had made ignoring who she was growing inside me. From an outsider's perspective, I likely appeared overbearing, intense, and maybe even selfish, but in that moment and at that time, nothing else mattered except for me and my baby. I was obsessed with becoming the perfect mom who did everything right.

Thus, this was our new life. I was the leader of our little team, in charge of making decisions on how to raise this baby. I mean, it made sense. I had the knowledge base. *I spent one hundred and ten percent of my time with her, I should know best, right?* But what happens when you don't know something you *should* know, and you feel alone? What happens when you dive into the deep end with a baby who doesn't sleep and cries for many hours of the day? When everyone around you seems to have their sh*t together and you feel the pressure to hold it all together? When you are highly educated on the subject of small humans, except all you do is bounce on exercise balls and say "shh" for hours of the day to get a

nap in and keep on schedule? I was losing control—control of the anxiety, control of myself, control of the entire situation. Knowledge didn't
seem to matter. There was conflicting advice in every book I read. I felt
alone, no one knew my child better than I did, but did I really *know* her?
Self-doubt followed the overwhelming amount of information overdose
and loneliness because no one else seemed to admit that they had no
idea what they were doing. What an isolating motherhood I was living.

Despite these feelings, we were making it through. Adrenaline is an
amazing thing. I survived—we survived—the first one hundred days. But
we had hardly any sleep. I know people say that you learn to function
on a small amount of sleep when you have a baby, but I was functioning
on NO sleep. When I wasn't reading about infant development, sleep
patterns, breastfeeding, and developmental leaps, I was tending to my
high-needs baby who had to be bounced to sleep day and night, nursed
nine thousand times a day (and night), and didn't like to be put down
for very long. I thought, *I should be able to do this, everyone else does.* This
attitude resulted in exhaustion beyond exhaustion, really. I sat in my
nursing chair at night and googled the closest hotel, dreaming of lying
in a really soft bed and sleeping for as long as I wanted—uninterrupted
sleep with NO chance of being woken. I had developed anxiety around
sleep—I knew I needed to sleep, but as soon as my head hit the pillow,
I became scared of having to deal with my baby when she woke again,
which perpetuated the cycle of sleeplessness and exhaustion. I am sure I
could have been hospitalized at this point. I wished I had been. This is
where the downward spiral started. The anxiety and exhaustion turned
into anger and depression; I had yet to feel true joy in this experience.
Instead, it all felt overwhelming. I knew I needed to tackle the sleep
issues first—I needed it, and we needed it as a family. I just felt lost and,
more importantly, guilty. Having heard and seen all the mom-shaming

on the topic of sleep and knowing that every mom I knew at this point co-slept or didn't believe in sleep training, I felt insecure and wasn't sure which direction to move in.

On an early spring day, four months into my daughter's life, I was walking with her in the carrier, hoping she would nap. I was obsessed with keeping a nap schedule. It was the same route I always walked, but on this day I started to move toward an overpass nearby. Over and over again, I crossed this overpass. I don't know why, but it kept drawing me in. There was something freeing about it. I wondered if I would be better off if I just jumped—it was as though the idea of jumping welcomed me with open arms, telling me to finally get the rest my body so desperately craved. It made me feel supported, like if I leaned in and finally let go, I would be completely supported, weightless, and free. I would feel free—free from guilt and judgment, free from my obsessions, and free from anxiety and the constant chaos in my mind and around me. *Oh, how beautiful it would be to just be free from all of that.* What a terrifying thought. *What type of person thinks this? What type of mother, who SO badly wanted a child, would have these thoughts?* I walked home with tears pouring down my face. I sat on my couch, defeated and exhausted. My husband came home to a hysterical mess. I remember telling him I was miserable, that I couldn't and didn't want to do this anymore. I needed sleep. I needed a break. Motherhood shouldn't feel this way. My baby was exhausted, and so was I. I needed to get us sleeping, but like every mom out there, I often felt unsure and just wanted to do what was best for her. This is the first time I listened to my intuition and made the choice that I knew would work for MY family.

We implemented our sleep-training strategies and our little girl proved to be a strong-willed baby. Hearing my baby cry was hard, but I knew we needed better rest and quality sleep to be a happy family. To show up fully as the mother I wanted to be, I knew I needed better rest. My baby is so wanted, so loved, so cared for, and although hearing her cry broke my heart, it also saved my life. I kept our sleep training a secret from most people for a while because I felt like a failure during that time. I knew it was best for my family, but I just couldn't understand why I wasn't like other moms. I was so worried about what other people would think; this fear of judgment consumed me like high school drama.

I saw people reach out on online mommy groups asking about sleep training and many of the responses were judgmental. Mom-shaming was, and is, an actual thing! I read the messages and could tell these moms felt like I did—unsure, judged for their choice, and desperate for rest! I couldn't bear to see these mamas, who were clearly struggling and looking for support, receive judgment instead. I thought, *what if we could all provide nonjudgmental support? What if we could all be the biggest cheerleaders for one another? Shouldn't motherhood feel more like a tribe and less like we are fighting to sit at the cool table at lunchtime?*

So I started sharing . . . sharing my struggle with anger, frustration, depression, and anxiety. I shared how I knew what I needed to do, but I held back because I was scared of what others might think. I shared how I thought I was going to be a *perfect* mama but instead felt inadequate in every way. I decided that if telling my story, if being truthful, open, and honest could help just ONE person feel less alone, then I needed to do that. The surprising part was that once I started sharing my story, I was the one who felt less alone. In sharing my knowledge, my failures, and my triumphs, I created my community and found my tribe. I knew I needed to do something more. I knew I had so much more to give to mothers and families now as a nurse and as a woman, and I needed to find my way. Thus, along came The Mama Coach. Just before my daughter's first birthday, I launched The Mama Coach in Vancouver, Canada—my way of helping mothers, one by one, find their way through the chaotic and sleepless first year of motherhood. As a sleep consultant and a lactation consultant, I get the privilege of joining mamas in their homes and providing that support they need to make a change in their life!

Prior to becoming a mama myself, all I saw was the birth of a baby in my labor rooms. Now, however, I know it is so much more than that—it is also the birth of a mother. The mother needs to be nurtured and cared for just as much as a newborn. Mothers need encouragement, support, and education without the judgment or the pressure to feel like they need to do everything perfectly. I wish someone had said to me, "*You* are the one person who can give your children a happy mother and, in the end, that's all that matters. Babies don't care if they are breastfed or bottle fed, they don't care if they are sleep trained or co-sleep, they don't care if they have an ideal schedule or sleep whenever they want. What they want and what they need is a healthy, present mama who loves them unconditionally." For me, this was not an easy realization; it took many months of feeling lost and trying to find "perfection" to finally listen to my instincts and to do what worked for our family. I can promise you this: No matter what, your baby is SO loved, motherhood is SO hard, but **you've got this, Mama!**

Only when you quiet the chaos within, will you be attuned to the peaceful whispers within you.

~ Tania Jane Moraes-Vaz
@theholisticwarriorlife

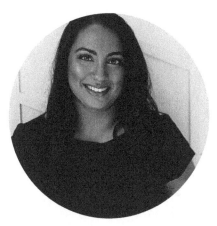

Tania Jane Moraes-Vaz

Tania is a woman of many capes—wife to a wonderful man who is her rock and love, mom to an intuitive and spirited three-year-old son, a creative maven, and a visionary at heart. Tania is a multi-best-selling author, founder of her two brands—The Holistic Warrior Life Co and Warrior Life Creative Co, and host of *The Holistic Warrior Life Podcast.*

She graduated with a BA in English Literature and Creative Writing from the University of Waterloo and found her way back to this soul-calling through a series of "yes"-ventures in the world of writing and publishing. Being avidly passionate about holistic health and healing, plus being confronted with her own health diagnosis of polycystic ovarian syndrome (PCOS) eight years ago, drove her down the rabbit hole of all things holistic health. She is now a certified Reiki Master (RM) and NLP coach and a soon-to-be certified holistic nutritionist.

An entrepreneur at heart, Tania knew deep within that she was not meant for the corporate grind and needed to live a life by design. Her PCOS diagnosis and her journey into motherhood almost three years ago catalyzed her first steps into what would become a multi-faceted business that merged all her passions together—visual art, writing, and mentorship—to help women express themselves.

Ⓦ theholisticwarriorlife.com

🄾 @theholisticwarriorlife

🅕 taniajanemoraesvaz

~ To my son Arnold-Aedan: Mama loves you many. Thank you for being my greatest teacher. My hubby, Alan, thank you for being my mirror and rock. My soul sisters (you know who you are), thank you for seeing me, all of me.

Nine

SELF-AWARE IS THE NEW BLACK
Tania Jane Moraes-Vaz

*"She was the kind of person who took care of
things by herself. She'd never ask anybody for
advice or help. It wasn't a matter of pride, I
think. She just did what seemed natural to her."*

- Haruki Murakami

A good friend of mine, Sarah Swain, once said, "Your entire life can
change in a year, but only *if* you let it." I initially heard this proclamation
at her very first women's empowerment summit that I had the fortune of
attending last September. Out of that entire weekend with its powerful
lineup of speakers, it was this nugget of wisdom that I carried close to
my heart. It is only this year that I realized how that one mantra guided
my entire year since then and how things unfolded in all categories—the
good, the not so good, and the "my life is over." Let's unpack a bit and
go on a soul-venture.

Warning: *Some of this information may be triggering, but I
encourage you to read on with an open mind and heart and sit
with whatever feelings surface.*

You see, this time last year I felt like I was on a precipice—fight or flee. Live or die. And boy, did I come close to that very last option—die—last year, not once but three times. And the year before that, at least a few times. The year prior to that, a few other times. For as long as I can remember, I have struggled with depression, anxiety, and post-traumatic stress disorder (PTSD). Growing up, I didn't have these names for my feelings and out-of-body experiences, but I felt them coursing through me—my face heating up, my hands clammy and trembling ever so slightly but not noticeably, that pit in my stomach growing deeper and deeper, my heart rate pounding faster than a sledgehammer, all sound around me muffled, my stance slowly shrinking inward causing drooping shoulders, my voice softening and quieting until it's not even a whisper but a muffled cry: *Girl, that fight didn't last too long. I'm tired, T. Can we call it a day and go to our safe space now?* My body feels heavy, yet weightless, knowing that I'm not fully there anymore. I have completely stepped out of it. I have dissociated with it, yet I am still tethered to it, to their noise, to the chaos, to their insults. I feel every physical lash and punch, but mentally and emotionally, I'm not there. *You must not be seen or heard, Tania. This is the only way. There, you're safe now. Look, your body is down there, nobody can hurt you now. You can go back when you feel it's safe.* Every single time. Every time a boundary was crossed. Every time a hand hit me, every time a threat was made, and every time I had to experience yelling, manipulation and, in one case, sexual assault in my first year of university (thank God that I somehow managed to wake up, scream, and fight my way out of that dark place, literally and figuratively).

I won't dive into the dark, sordid details of my past, but such was my life growing up, all the way into my early years of university. I didn't realize that fight or flee had become a pattern for me, a way of life: a pattern ingrained in me since I was a child, further perpetuated by every experience. Most days I'd choose to fight, but there were some days where I'd completely flee and hide. It was my default programming (some days it still is) until I decided I would no longer let it dictate my life and debilitate me. Choosing to *fight* for myself—to be seen and heard—and advocate for myself has been a lesson I have been learning my whole life—sometimes through traumatic experiences growing up, other times through a health diagnosis; sometimes through the loss of misaligned job opportunities and business partnerships, other times through some heart-wrenching breakups with people who weren't meant for me. I wish I could tell you that I have mastered everything, but that would be a lie. What I now know is that I have a set of healing tools I can use to ground myself, stand strong within myself and, of course, advocate for myself no matter the kind of chaos rampant around me.

The biggest test of this "mastery" is motherhood—not just the physical changes and challenges it brings but also the mental and emotional. I knew that given my PCOS diagnosis and my childhood trauma, I was at a higher risk of slipping into postpartum depression. I just underestimated exactly how deep that spiral would be. Well, let's say that the spiral lasted two long, nightmarish years, and for the most part I was physically present as a mom, but emotionally and mentally, I felt so alone and checked out. My saving grace? God, and through him, my baby's kisses and giggles, his smile and that look of admiration and love, and those itty-bitty hands touching my face whenever I was sad, seemingly or visibly. This spiral ended at the beginning of this year. Last year, however, was a different story.

After staying home on maternity leave for almost a year and half and caring for my little boy through his personal health battles, I returned to working full time at the bank contact center last February. I did so in hopes of alleviating the financial stress placed on our family by my extended leave. I did so because I needed the human interaction. And moreover, I did so because I didn't quite have clarity in who I am, what makes me, well, me, and I wasn't speaking my truth or living it (*although I wasn't aware of the latter part at the time*). It's amazing how sometimes trauma will guide your steps if you let it, only to find yourself in more trauma as time progresses. When I first started working there, our training schedules were 9:00 to 5:00, which was quite an adjustment for me with a young baby in tow, but I got'er done! Eventually we had to pick our shift schedules, and guess what I chose? 6:00 p.m. to 3:00 a.m. Crazy, right? In hindsight, I cannot believe I put my mind and body through that wringer, but at the time, I was super excited—excited to get away from home and be on an opposite schedule as everyone else, excited to have my space, excited for the flexibility. Also, the extra money didn't hurt. I thought it would help calm and pacify my already emotionally frail and combative marriage—and it did, for a while at least. I loved the team and the work culture, and I am still in touch with some of my colleagues. But boy did those overnight hours do me in.

I didn't clue in until August last year that by taking on those work hours, what I was doing was actually hiding: hiding from the conflict in my marriage, hiding from taking ownership for my wants, needs, and desires, hiding from the success I craved, hiding from my soul-calling purpose. And so I continued to hide, plastering a smile on my face and fighting the anxiety and depressive episodes that still ran rampant through my body. My home was very much crowded with nonstop unannounced visitors, and physical and emotional boundaries continued to be crossed. Additionally, the one person in my life who I counted on to listen to me and see me, like really listen to what I *wasn't* saying out loud and really see what I was trying to mask all along (*Hi, I'm here. I need to be seen. I need to be held. Hi, can I get a kiss, babe? Can I get a hug, babe? It's been so long since we've hugged or kissed. Hi, I'm here, the woman you fell in love with. I'm still in here. It feels so heavy. All I want is peace. Calm. Understanding. Joy.*) was miles apart from me emotionally, though we were physically present with each other. I mean, if anyone looked in— unless they really knew me or what was going on—they would assume I had a picture-perfect life. Home, check. Married, check. Has a child, check. Happy, unchecked. In love, unchecked. Appreciated, unchecked. Loved, probably—the forecast just looks a bit gloomy right now thanks to the responsibilities of #adultlife #momlife. And so the cycle continued until midsummer when I felt the cloud settle on me bit by bit. I would speak my truth and take one step forward, only to take ten steps back. I kept pushing my mental, emotional, and physical fatigue and stress to the back burner. I muffled my voice and suppressed my truth back into my throat and down into my heart and gut. I ignored my intuition. I ignored all the signs telling me I wasn't happy or fulfilled. There is more to life than constantly combating with your spouse and living in an empty marriage or a marriage rampant with if/then conditions. There is more to life than listening to the insults of perfect strangers over the phone, all over a particular bank policy they don't agree with. And there certainly is more to life than living your life tiptoeing around the opinions, likes, and dislikes of everyone else. Argh. *Guess who's back, T? Me. I'm here to stay in the limelight. You tried suppressing me this year, but it's not working, face it. I will keep coming back until you decide enough is enough.* Before I knew it, I had tears streaming down my face at 3:30 a.m. for no reason at all. I had tears on my way home from work as well as at other times like when I'd stand in my kitchen with the lights off since everyone was asleep. Before I knew it, I was sick. Always sick, all the damn time. And guess what? Motherhood doesn't give you time off, not all the time at least.

I always tell my clients that what we don't heal and address emotionally manifests itself psychosomatically. Suffice it to say that keeping my truth to myself, dimming my light, and playing puppet to everyone else's expectations of me resulted in me getting sick with four ear and throat infections, one severe case of strep throat, and adrenal failure (yes, that's right, especially after I spent years healing it). Oh, that case of strep throat was the final straw. That was September 21, 2018. A few weeks prior to me contracting strep throat, I had locked myself in my en suite bathroom where I wrote good-bye letters to each of the people I was close to in my life. My next step was to just do the damn thing: rid myself of this pain I could no longer bear inside me, for good this time. Then a shrill cry and a constant rat-a-tat on the bathroom door jolted me awake from that trance. *Oh, sweet Lord. God bless my baby boy.* "Mama, where are you? Mama, you sadh (sad)? Mama, I love you. Mama, come out. Maman." His cry and his voice brought me back to myself, to my very earthly body. I felt fully merged with myself. That out-of-body experience snapped like a cord that was at its breaking point. Notebook down. Pen down. Exacto knife down and tucked away safely, my left wrist carrying traces of what I would have done had my son's cries not woken me from that very hypnotic trance. But I never dare speak this truth out loud to anyone in my household except for a few trusted sisters in my life—and my counselor, of course.

About two weeks after I recovered from strep throat, I gave my notice at work and bid them a bittersweet farewell. My resignation only seemed to aggravate those in my closest ecosystem even more because they didn't understand my reasoning, not because there was no love there. "How can you leave a steady, stable job? You should have pushed through it. You think you're the only one with health issues, fertility challenges, depression? What makes you so special?" Such were the things said to me in the aftermath of that choice.

I won't drone on and on, but after that overnight stint, I went to work for my ex-publisher on a full-time contract basis. Grateful as I was for the opportunity, something didn't sit well energetically, not anymore at least. There was that pit again. Those feelings. Those out-of-body experiences, usually after my phone dinged with a text or email notification. But I ignored those intuitive nudges. I was angry, irritated, burned out, and all-out horrible to people in my life, all because I couldn't ask for what I wanted in this particular contract opportunity, all because I was living so out of alignment with myself. Well, that opportunity came to an end earlier this year, abruptly, aggressively, and traumatically on many fronts, especially the personal one. Remember when I said trauma has a way of informing you about what you like or don't like and, of course, when you are living in alignment with yourself or not. I kid you not, no sooner did that opportunity end that it felt like a giant vacuum or void was created in my life. This void is how I realized that I had hidden behind that particular opportunity and what it represented to me: being seen, being heard, being acknowledged in some manner—something that was very much missing in my personal life.

The loss of that business partnership, while shitty at first, proved to be the healing salve for my two years of postpartum depression. It made me aware that I am worthy. It made me aware that I am enough just the way I am. It made me aware of the fact that I am a healer, I am an intuitive being, I am worthy of living my desires and asking for them. We all are, Mama. So please don't ever stop asking for them. It made me aware of the fact that my mind and intentions are powerful. My words, even more powerful. The way my environment and the people around me can impact me? Powerful. But I have a choice in that matter that is even more powerful—it is the secret sauce to changing your life. I became aware that I had choice all along. I simply had to take the first step. My life could change and would change, but only if I let it.

And so, with the help of a few trusted sisters/mamas, including my own, I have spent this past year re-parenting myself, mothering my very malnourished soul, and filling my own cup, unapologetically this time around. With the help and cooperation of my spouse, we have been actively working on our marriage—I am standing my ground more and more in our dynamic and being unapologetic with my pursuit of my dreams, and he now offers alternative suggestions and kicks my behind to show up when I can't (it wasn't always like this, that I can tell you). My son is growing to be an intuitive child who sometimes asks the silliest but most profound questions. He is my biggest teacher. But these changes didn't happen overnight. It took me taking the first step by advocating for myself—by leaving unaligned jobs, friendships, family relationships, and more. If it doesn't feel good, it has got to go. And no, I'm not talking about the hard things or the things that seem annoying but need to get done. I'm referring to the things we force—people, opportunities, places. Look at that "force" or resistance as a sign from your intuition asking you to wake up. Something is unaligned, and you need to act quickly. And if you ever feel backed into a corner like I did, please, please, ask for help or speak to a professional. Speak to someone who will listen. Know that you are never alone. Help is there all around us, be it through this book, online, or in person. Speak to yourself with kindness, with compassion, with grace, with love. Hug yourself gently first thing in the morning. Feel your face, feel your body, bring that awareness back to your breath. Use this practice whenever you are faced with situations that make you want to flee, mentally or emotionally. Stay grounded and anchored in who you are—as a woman, as a mama, and as a wife. When in doubt, lean on a trusted sister. When in doubt, if it doesn't feel good, no matter how hard you analyze it or how hard you try, simply take a deep breath in and release the person or opportunity with love. Your mental and emotional health are so very important. Nothing and no one should ever be prioritized over that. You cannot pour from an empty cup, and you cannot continue to eat from a plate that keeps overflowing. There needs to be a balance, even within the beautiful chaos that is motherhood. There still needs to be *you*. As you are. In your wholeness. Look in the mirror and repeat this out loud: "You've got this, Mama. Yes, you. You're amazing, you're worthy, you're beautiful, and you have every right to take up space, to speak your truth, and to do it unapologetically. You've got this, you always have."

You can choose
pain and
suffering, or you
can choose to
change.

~Mona Sharma
@monasharma

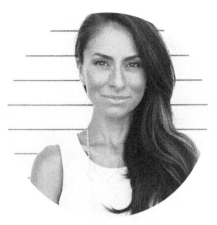

Mona Sharma

Mona Sharma is a thought leader and entrepreneur in the health and wellness industry. As a celebrity wellness educator who recently appeared on the Red Table Talk as Will Smith's holistic nutritionist and mind/body coach, she is also the founder of Xicama™, an innovative line of functional food and beverage products that deliver the gut- and immune-boosting benefits of the superfood Jicama.

Mona's early years were spent living on an ashram while learning of the power of food as medicine, yoga, and meditation to heal the body. After overcoming two heart surgeries, experiencing chronic anxiety, and burning out in the corporate world, she returned to her Ayurvedic roots and began her own healing journey, healing herself from the inside out. As a result, she takes a holistic view while partnering with functional medicine doctors to optimize each person's unique constitution.

Today Mona lives in Los Angeles where these are the pillars of her philosophy, helping her clients achieve their goals for long-term optimal health. She believes in functional nutrition as medicine, breath and movement as therapy, and meditation as mind reconditioning, ridding the effects of learned behavior, stress, and inflammation of the body. Mona awakens the health, mindset, and lifestyle that allow her clients to thrive.

 monasharma.com

MonaSharmaWellness

@monasharma

~Elijah and India, thank you for making my once-broken heart beam with love greater than I could ever imagine. I adore you, and I'm so blessed to be your mama. To my husband, Craig, you are my greatest love and supporter. I love you. And to my parents, thank you for loving me through all the challenges and for guiding me to my true calling in this lifetime.

Ten

AWAKENING
Mona Sharma

"You are in a position, starting now, to adopt the role of self-healer. By going deeper into the power of awareness, you can activate the hidden potential of the healing system that you already depend upon every day. We hope this all sounds exciting, because some major life changes lie ahead."

–Deepak Chopra

I was twenty-one years old when I woke up in the hospital the morning after my second heart surgery for ongoing heart palpitations that left me feeling faint. The surgery didn't work. I was given the option to live with a pacemaker my whole life or live with my palpitations. Obviously, I chose the latter. I had been conscious for the whole procedure, watching my heart on a massive monitor with wires in my chest as they injected me with different meds—all with the aim to induce an "episode." This time during the surgery all I could do was cry and wonder what I had ever done to my body to end up here and *why* I would agree to such an invasive procedure again. I think I had gotten used to living with the label of "heart problem," living on meds, and living in an invisible bubble while shielding myself from all that life had to offer—yet wanting all of it. I strongly identified as someone who functioned with a victim mentality. So the idea of surgery, AKA someone trying to fix me quickly without me having to do the work around healing, seemed appealing. I disregarded any possibility of alternative healing, and most certainly, I was completely disconnected from my intuition and the possibility of loving or healing myself first.

My heart palpitations started almost immediately after waking up that morning. Stress was a pretty common trigger, and I'm sure this episode was likely the aftershock of all the meds leaving my body that my heart had to process. I was alone, and I broke down in tears because having this heart condition meant I was going to continue living life declaring I had a heart issue with the side effects of medications that made me lethargic, uninspired, and overweight. And I did not want to be lethargic, uninspired, and overweight.

I know that things could have been worse. I could have had cancer or another disease. Or I could have died. But I think each person's version of illness or trauma is all they know. And in my world, I was suffering and sad, and this meant I was living life associating with suffering and sadness.

This period was an all-time low for me. My parents had recently divorced after thirty-five years of marriage, and my mother and I were adjusting to a new way of living together. Although we could see the upside of their decision, there was tremendous sadness and a jarring divide within my family. I'm not sure how my mother held it together. She was so strong through it all, and I never saw a tear. We were the type of family that never talked about our feelings. We took pride in wearing the "stiff upper lip," and so we repressed it all. To top it off, I had also broken up with my best friend, who had become my boyfriend, who I had clung to for stability even though it was a terrible relationship. I was about to graduate university majoring in Art History with absolutely no clue what I was going to do for a career. I had fast-tracked just about everything growing up because of my much-older siblings, and I frankly thought that they (adults) had it so much easier. Lesson learned. I was sad, stressed, lost, and now sick. But the only option I knew was to muscle through it, to pretend everything was fine, and to keep moving forward. *Sound familiar?*

Although life put a lot of great gifts in front of me during my twenties, it was certainly the toughest decade of my life. I somehow ended up working in the corporate beauty world as a sales and artistry trainer and really thought I had nailed what was going to make me happy: sexy-sounding job, a great salary, opportunities to travel and work with celebrities, and access to high fashion (this is where everyone's eyes light up). But once the novelty and excitement passed, the reality of having a typical corporate sales job kicked in—working long hours, accepting recognition based on numbers, eating out all the time, waking up alone in many different cities, being away from family and routine, and facing lots of inauthenticity with the relationships I had because I was playing the role. My boss at the time was controlling and often verbally abusive, and the type of person who when she was feeling bad made sure the people around her felt just as bad. I was an easy target back then. I endured it because I didn't have the courage to stand up for myself. A person who plays victim doesn't believe in herself and has strong feelings of guilt, shame, and unworthiness. I was able to play a role and step into the person I thought others wanted to see. However, inside, the reality of who I was didn't match up with all that I portrayed myself to be. Also, how could I feel happy when the person I wanted to be didn't align with the low vibration I was feeling and living with daily? I felt like I had two parts of me constantly at war with each other, each one doing a one-two-step dance.

As a result, my heart palpitations were in full effect, I was overweight, I stopped getting my periods, I cried every other day, and I smoked and drank regularly (yep, smoking with a heart condition) because my mindset was in survival mode, which I hid well. I burned out. Every day I desperately asked the Universe for a sign for what I was supposed to be doing, for change, and for guidance. The fact was that the sign was always right in front of me. At some point I learned how to live out of alignment with happiness. I could see the end goal and feeling I wanted, but I had no clue *how* to get there. It is said that people or experiences come into your life for a reason to help you learn or grow—I see now that this experience and my boss were gifts that changed it all.

I booked a vacation a few months in advance, deciding to get myself back to the ashram where my parents took our family when I was growing up. Traditionally, ashram living means practicing daily meditation, yoga, and chanting. There is a focus on eating healing Ayurvedic meals and relaxing to heal and connect to self (or God). My father, being from India, was familiar with this tradition and likely felt the call to return for similar reasons as I did—to unplug. He also knew it would benefit my mother who has suffered from a debilitating autoimmune disease for as long as I can remember. I spent my summers at the ashram as a child, and it felt like torture at the time—what kid wants to get up at 5:00 a.m. to meditate and do yoga and eat veggies nonstop? In looking back however, these summers laid the foundation for who I was to become. I saw firsthand the healing power of food with my mother's disease, the evident stress relief, and the transformative effects of yoga and meditation.

It felt like we could exhale. I grew up with this awareness so I'm not too sure why I didn't return to the ashram sooner, but I finally listened to the voice inside that told me I had to go back "home."

It had probably been about seven years since I'd been to the ashram. I can actually say that this upcoming visit was the one decision that changed everything because I was saying yes to putting myself first again. As a result and in preparation, I started to take note of the food I was eating that made me feel awful. I started working with a holistic psychotherapist. I started exercising and became the friend who tried to make the healthy choice. And then, shortly after I booked this trip and decided to focus on my health and happiness, I met the love of my life completely out of the blue on a freelance makeup job. He was the director on set that day. I'll never forget leaving for my trip a few weeks after we started dating. My heart felt open again, and it was one of the best trips of my life. I was able to sit in deep meditation, acknowledge the necessity of daily gratitude, practice self-love and self-care, and be in a community of like-minded people who also wanted to feel good and just exhale again. There is a lot of free time with no TVs, phones, or computers around, so I used the trip as an opportunity to purge all the toxic emotions, thoughts, stories, and events from my mind and body. I was done with the past and the constant blame of myself, and I promised myself that I would never ignore my spirit or my heart again. Now was the time to return to love.

There is power in self-compassion and self-care. I took a step back from the cold impression I had of myself and recognized that my suffering was a learned behavior used to repress what I was feeling. Having mindfulness around self-judgment and pain allows you to make better decisions because you see clearly what hurts and what is hard, when in reality, you are the controller. You can choose pain and suffering, or you can choose to change. I chose change, which means I chose me again. Now I had a partner who had my back and encouraged me to follow what feels good. Shortly after this island trip, I moved in with Craig, quit my nasty job and toxic habits, and began my journey in the health and wellness industry. I went back to the ashram, became a yoga teacher, and then soon after, a registered holistic nutritionist to use food as medicine as well as a neuro-linguistic programming (NLP) coach to help my clients unlearn some of the programming that no longer served them. When my training happened, my father gave me the greatest compliment of all. He said, "The vibration of the ashram never left you." I just had to learn how to recognize everything that I didn't want before I could see everything that I did.

Trust the journey.

The greatest and most important adventure of our lives is discovering who we really are. In yoga and meditation, one of the questions we're taught to ask is "Who am I?" Yet so many of us experience life not really knowing. We're disconnected, and we often get used to living in disconnect—from our bodies, our sense of self, and even from our intuition, which is there to guide us to live well. Instead, we tune in to our awful inner critic that feeds us all the wrong ideas and information about ourselves. It's a loud voice, isn't it? The one that talks you out of feeling too good, the one that can make you feel awful about yourself, and the one that even talks you out of creating habits to change your life because it says you might fail. I call this "spinning" with my clients. When we get to a point when fear, sadness, pain, anxiety, or worry feel like too much, we spin so fast, like on a carousel at an amusement park, that we can't stop.

Repeated and persistent negative thoughts over time become you. Just like food is information for our cells, the power of our thoughts is information as well. Every cell in your body begins to listen and believe these negative thoughts that fuel physical imbalance and dis"ease." For me, I was sending myself consistent thoughts including, "I'm not happy. What's the point? I'm sick. It's too hard. I'm tired. I have no energy." *How on earth would my body heal with this mantra?* Low-vibration thoughts bring low-vibration energy—it's no wonder I was attracting so much of what I didn't want at that time. We know our mind is powerful, yet we give no attention to tuning in to see if the thoughts themselves are fueling us or depleting us or whether they're even true.

The answer when asked "Who am I?" should be a collection of descriptive words including healthy, vibrant, energetic, go-getter, self-healer, powerful, and joyful. Our bodies should be flooding with endorphins to match. Science has proven that simply recalling memories of positive emotions can be just as powerful as an actual event stimulating the response. You can try it right now—close your eyes and think about a time in your life when you felt happy, at peace, healthy, or even joyful. Get clear on the memory and what you felt like in your body at that time. Take a picture of it in your mind with as much detail as possible so you can always recall it when you're feeling down or unhappy or sick. It's up to us to use our minds and thought power as tools, even on the days we struggle.

It's no surprise that most of my clients today have started with me to lose weight, gain energy, get a six-pack, or do a headstand, etc. However, they stay with me because I'm able to guide them to feeling inner peace and happiness and self-compassion to heal. To my point above about thought power, positive affirmations are great, but they'll only work if your *belief* matches the power of your thoughts. As I learned, I had to start *believing* that I could be healthy, happy, and energetic before any changes would stick. I had to hit rock bottom to make the necessary changes, but really, the decision to change can happen at any point or even every day for that matter. So with my clients, through consistent practice, I support them in turning down the noise of the inner critic and self-limiting beliefs and guide them to rediscover what it feels like to live with a happy mind and body. The side effect of this rediscovery is that it can actually turn off any physical symptoms in the body—things like physical pain, digestive issues, and hormone imbalance because you take the body out of feeling chronic stress and suffering into feeling good, even if it means recalling a memory of a time of feeling good. If you can recall it or dream it, you can become it; your circumstances and your genetics do not determine your destiny.

I wish the doctors had asked me about my stress levels, about my diet, about my happiness, or even about what was happening in my life at the time my heart palpitations were at their worst. But they didn't. Surgery was the fastest, easiest solution, and like I said, who doesn't want the fastest solution? Don't get me wrong; we need doctors and medications and surgery, but I'm beyond proud to be part of the paradigm shift that is happening in the world of wellness today—to support each individual by combining science and a whole mind/body/spirit point of view. We are so much more than our symptoms. I often partner with functional medicine doctors to address each person's unique constitution to get to the root cause of illness and imbalance in order to heal from the inside out. My protocol always includes food as medicine, movement as therapy, and mindfulness to recondition the mind and body to thrive.

Today I'm a mother to Elijah and baby India. Becoming a mother has been one of the most transformative events of my life, literally, because as mothers, we have to say good-bye to our sense of self and personal freedom. But it's also a constant opportunity to learn, forgive, let go, and choose to step into a better version of ourselves. I describe motherhood as the highest form of personal growth because now there are little ones absorbing our actions and our beliefs on every aspect of being. How can I be a better teacher and role model for them? Although my parents split up, it's crazy to think that they were my greatest teachers in leading to my career, success, and story. I'm reminded constantly of the decision I had to make to become healthy and happy. Today the challenges are different and my mindset is different, but every day is truly an opportunity to decide whether I'm going to stay the path of happiness and wellness or not. Remember, Mamas, the transformative effects of self-compassion are endless. Every decision either fuels your health and happiness or depletes you. Once you begin to embrace yourself wholly and develop a mindset to believe your health and destiny can be greater than you imagine, making the right decisions becomes easy because you always choose what nourishes you most.

Vulnerability frees us from our shame and insecurities and helps us realize we are all alike.

~Andrea Taylor
@a_real_canadian_housewife

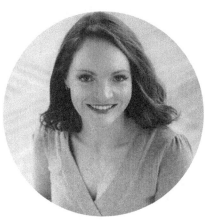

Andrea Taylor

Andrea never envisioned herself working in the health and wellness field. For many years she led an unhealthy, unhappy life fraught with severe mental health challenges. It was after spending much of her life in this lonely darkness that a quiet desperation for a change began to grow. Like a lotus flower that grows beneath the murky waters before blossoming into its true beauty, Andrea's desperation slowly blossomed into a newfound belief that there was something more out there for her. Andrea went on to transform herself from the inside out by developing and implementing her own holistic interventions. It was through this journey that she discovered and now pursues her heart's true purpose as a passionate mental health advocate and holistic health and wellness practitioner who works with women to uncover their own passions and purpose while living their happiest and healthiest lives yet.

Andrea is a Certified Fitness Trainer, Corrective Exercise Specialist, Nutrition Coach, and Certified Transformation Specialist. She also specializes in pre- and postnatal health. Andrea has three amazing little girls with her handsome hubby, Justin. Running her coaching and network marketing businesses, while being home and present for her girls, fills her cup every day. Andrea understands the challenges women face as mothers and loves helping moms redefine and rediscover themselves again beyond their title "Mom." She wants every mom to know they are never alone; they deserve to feel powerful, worthy, and unbloodystoppable.

Andrea may have transformed from suicidal to a woman empowered, but at the end of the day, she is just a real Canadian housewife.

Ⓦ   tayloredlifestyles.ca
f   arealcanadianhousewife
Ⓘ   @a_real_canadian_housewife

*~Mom, thank you for being my greatest cheerleader, my friend, the reflection in the mirror when I needed it, and for teaching me what it means to be a mom. Because you always did, I, too, finally **BELIEVE.** Justin, thank you for loving not only my light but my darkness and for giving me something I could never live without.*

*And for the pieces of my heart and soul: Ayla, Ashlyn, and Brielle—know how incredibly special you are **just** as you are. I know the footprints you leave in this world will be everlasting, no matter your path, for you have already left footprints on the hearts of everyone around you. With every part of my being, I thank you. You truly brought me to life. I love you to infinity and beyond . . . and back again!*

Eleven

MEMOIRS OF A REAL CANADIAN HOUSEWIFE
Andrea Taylor

"Like the lotus flower that is born out of mud, we must honor the darkest parts of ourselves and the most painful of our life's experiences, because they are what allow us to birth our most beautiful self."
~Debbie Ford

Being a mom is wonderful, isn't it? We love our children—they give us purpose and add new meaning to our lives. Everything feels blissful once we hold these tiny little beings, these extensions of ourselves. There is nothing like seeing your baby for the first time—suddenly your heart fills up with this unwavering, unconditional love you never knew existed. Life is perfect, right?! The problem is that there is another side to motherhood no one talks about: a darker, lonelier, isolating side; a side so wrought with feelings of shame, guilt, overwhelm. A darkness that many of us are completely unprepared for. Some days are bright, wonderful, and filled with so much love, while other days feel as though we are in a deep, dark, winding tunnel with no light at the end. Some days we don't even know what the hell we are feeling. But wait, we are supposed to be nothing but ecstatic, right? And we are ecstatic. We are happy beyond our wildest dreams . . . yet sometimes underneath our newfound love and elation something else is quietly growing, its claws sinking into us ever so softly but ever so surely—exhaustion, overwhelm, self-doubt, and isolation. We begin to harbor feelings of sadness, inadequacy, insecurity, and guilt. Oh, that fucking mom guilt. Oh, how that mom guilt can make us question everything we are and have ever done: Am *I* a good mom? Am *I* doing enough? Am *I* enough? It is so bloody *hard!* My mom has always joked that when we are handed that beautiful baby, we are also unknowingly handed a lifetime of guilt and self-doubt. Motherhood, in all its glory and overwhelming love, brings stress, frustration, shame, insecurities, feelings of inadequacy, anxiety, depression, exhaustion, and sleep deprivation (yes, these are the same things, but let's be honest: sleep is a distant memory to many of us). Motherhood becomes an all-encompassing and never-ending cycle of taking care of everyone else and ensuring everyone else's needs are met. Before we even realize it, we become second-class citizens in our own lives. We feel guilty for everything we do or don't do and compare ourselves to virtually everyone. We judge ourselves, which often leads to judging others . . . we enter a crazy cyclone of judgment and then feel shitty about ourselves. We lose a sense of who we are, our worthiness, and our wants and needs. When do we start being kind to ourselves again? When are we allowed to feel important again? When do we grant ourselves some grace? When are we allowed to talk about the aspects of motherhood that make us feel shame and guilt? And most importantly, when do we start giving ourselves a pat on the back, acknowledging the amazing job we really are doing? Because I promise you, Mama, you are doing a far better job than you realize.

I wonder when we became a culture where, as moms, we only have (or are willing to share) two motherhood personalities? The first is a perfect

self/family image where life is great—our inner *Mary Poppins.* The second
is a frustrated, hot mess of a mom where we joke about needing a glass of
wine at 10:00 a.m. because it's already been "that kind of day." When did
we become a culture where expressing how we feel means we are seen as
crazy, emotional, overly sensitive, or irrational? Why can't we just be real
and vulnerable? Why can't we just cut the bullshit? If you have ever had
moments where you feel like you are ready to fall apart, scream, cry, or
just want to run away, can I get an AMEN?! I sure have, and to be honest,
I have these feelings far more often than I care to admit. I think most of
us do. How often do you feel like you've lost a part of yourself, a part of
your identity outside of being "a mom?" Maybe you're beating yourself
up for not losing that baby weight or for not eating well or taking any
time for yourself (but of course, when you finally do, you feel guilty for
that too). So what do we do? We hide it, we get frustrated with our kids,
our husbands, and ourselves, we eat some yummy chocolate and wash it
down with a bottle of wine. We basically do whatever we can to numb
our feelings and avoid them. We do what we feel we need to do to "get
through." We share, superficially, that we are stressed because our kids are
driving us nuts, when deep down maybe we are stressed because we are
questioning our parenting . . . we are questioning ourselves, constantly
wondering whether we are doing a good enough job. *Could I be doing
more?* The reality is (and I hope I don't lose you here) that we CAN be
doing more, but not for others. We *can* show ourselves some compassion. We *can* bring some light, purpose, and identity back to ourselves
and who we are as a woman. We can detach for a few minutes from the
coveted title of "Mom" and make simple and incredibly positive choices
in our day-to-day life that will help us better "get through." So why don't
we? Well, change is hard. The truth is, it's easier to remain where we are
because it's comfortable, familiar, and safe. It's *normal* to struggle, and

yet admitting or even understanding the truth behind *why* we are truly struggling seems so hard. Motherhood can make the calmest, most *put-together* woman feel undone. For those of us who face challenges such as mental illness, this feeling of coming undone can become all-consuming. This is why having a support system is so crucial, and if you don't have a support system, ask your doctor for guidance to help with mental health struggles. It's okay to ask for help—it's not a sign of weakness, it's actually a sign of incredible strength and courage. You are not weak, Mama, and I see YOU.

I understand how hard it can be because I have been there. It was my own long, painful, dark, and scary journey with mental health that led me to the career I have today. Nutrition is one of the most crucial elements in creating and maintaining optimal mental well-being. I could reference countless papers and facts surrounding all the research that links nutritional deficiencies to an increased risk of depression and how our brains need omega fatty acids to help reduce inflammation—thus reducing our incidences and risks of anxiety—or how our brains are essentially incapable of functioning and firing properly without proper micro- and macro-nutrition on a regular basis.[1] For those who take any type of antidepressants or selective serotonin reuptake inhibitors (SSRIs), having a diet rich in wholesome fruits, vegetables, and omega fatty acids is imperative to ensure your medications are functioning optimally. Ever wonder why we are always hearing how important it is to eat foods high in antioxidants? It's to help rid our bodies of oxidation, AKA oxidative stress.[2] Our bodies are bombarded with toxins every day through our environment and the food we eat, thus creating oxidative stress in our bodies and brains and putting our brains at an increased risk of inflammation. Our quality of nutrition directly impacts the activity of our neurotransmitters, including serotonin, norepinephrine, and dopamine, all of which we need to feel happy and maintain optimal mental wellness. Antioxidants also help reduce the symptoms people experience when taking SSRIs, such as fatigue and constipation.[3] The reason I am passionate about educating moms on the importance of nutrition to help with our mental state (not to mention energy, ability to concentrate, immune health, cell health, etc.) is because not only did I turn to it as a crucial form of intervention in my own mental health treatment but I also saw how nutritional therapy helped my middle daughter fight back and transform from a newborn baby foaming at the mouth (who I rushed to the hospital) to a strong, spunky, and thriving three year old. So maybe before I go on, I should tell you a little bit more about my own journey.

Since my earliest memories, I always felt different. On the *outside,* it looked like I had a "normal" life. On the *inside,* however, I felt trapped and constantly tormented by my mind. I was first diagnosed with anxiety and depression and put on medication at seventeen years old. From there, my life spiraled out of control very quickly. I became consumed with self-hatred and felt so ashamed of who I was, but what seventeen year old knows who they are?! I felt like I wasn't good enough and not worthy of anything, and yes, this included life itself. I had a firm belief that I was a burden to everyone in my life. I began self-harming and eventually attempted suicide twice. For many years, that was my dark reality. I lost almost all my friends and made poor decisions, one after another, in a constant search for external validation. By the tender age of twenty-two, I was taking eleven pills a day. I didn't see a future for myself, nor did I feel deserving of one. I spent years in and out of therapy and lived an unbelievably unhealthy life. I was so unhappy and felt so hopeless. I felt apathetic at best. Anxiety and depression can feel as though you are in the depth of an eternal well with no light at the top. I remember getting to a point in my life where I thought that *there must be more to living life than this. I mean there has to be, right?* If there wasn't, I certainly didn't plan on sticking around much longer. I couldn't live that way anymore. I just fucking refused. That, right there, was a pivotal moment that completely changed the trajectory of my life. *That* was when I decided the pain of staying where I was was far more terrifying than the pain of taking a chance and making some changes. I started making a few small changes that eventually led to me transforming my life and ridding myself of all medication and those twenty-two pills!

Change can seem incredibly hard, but anyone is capable of doing it once they decide or realize that there is more to life than repeating the same cycle every single day. Afterall, Einstein did say the definition of insanity is doing the same thing repeatedly and expecting a different result, right? Now don't get me wrong. My transformation didn't happen overnight; it took years of small and consistent changes, but guess what? It worked! Something actually fucking worked. I began using nutrition and exercise as treatment interventions (along with personal development and therapy), and wow, was it ever worth it!

When I was pregnant with my firstborn, I prepared myself for post-partum depression because of course, given my history, I was a prime candidate for it. My daughter was born, and because I had already implemented small changes and healthy habits into my lifestyle, postpartum depression was something I sideswiped. *Yay me,* right? "Supermom" beating depression and anxiety again?! Well, life has a way of grounding us sometimes, and I was unprepared for a sudden move to a new city where I didn't know anyone followed by a miscarriage and D&C. Anyone who has lost a child during pregnancy will know it is a confusing sadness that catches you off guard. Life went on as did we, and luckily, we were blessed with another pregnancy. After the birth of our beautiful rainbow baby, I felt those baby blues slowly creeping in. But hey, that was no issue for this mental health warrior, right? At ten-days-old, my daughter woke up crying, and I got up with the thought that she was hungry. Within minutes, however, I realized she was barely breathing and was burning up. She could hardly open her eyes, and she started foaming at the mouth. Before I even knew what was happening, we were at the hospital. There were doctors and nurses everywhere—IV lines, oxygen tanks, sheer panic—just like in the movies. My world changed instantly. If you have ever had a sick child (or worse), it changes you in a very profound way. Our feisty and strong little girl fought like a champ and pulled through. I, on the other hand, was traumatized. Lack of sleep, extreme stress, poor nutrition, no exercise, being alone 99 percent of the time plus seeing nothing but hospital walls for two weeks caused my anxiety to spiral out of control. I slipped into severe postpartum depression. But wait, wasn't I the poster woman for mental health? Enter shame, frustration, and feeling like a fraud and failure.

My little girl was sick with a myriad of infections and was on anti-biotics and respiratory treatments for her first year of life. As soon as she was able to start solids, I did the only thing I knew—I used nutritional therapy to help rebuild her immune system. In just seven months, we were able to help her go from having a suppressed immune system to having normal blood markers. For anyone doubting the impact nutrition has on our immune response system and our body's ability to ward off illness and heal itself, I will tell you from the bottom of my heart that it *can* change and potentially save your life. Although my daughter's immune response system was no longer suppressed, my mental state *was*. Keeping ourselves and our little humans healthy and strong starts with having healthy cells. To help prevent cell damage, we need nutrients like beta-carotene, vitamin C, vitamin E, and omega fatty acids, all of which can be easily consumed through a wholesome, nutritious diet.[4]

I am now a mom to three incredible little girls, and like all moms, I continue to face new struggles and challenges. We each have our own struggles and past experiences that shape who we are and how we navigate motherhood. We are all just trying to do our best. With the influx of social media mom "support" groups (not always exactly supportive, am I right?), Google, how-to parenting books, and podcasts, we can find virtually anything right at our fingertips. For every website praising some specific method of parenting, there are five more dispelling the same theory. We live in a culture of new-age moms who are *supermoms* who do it all. But not just do it all . . . oh no, we *are expected and should* do it all: raise our kids, run a household, work, be on the parent council at school, volunteer, make fresh cookies for the bake sale, and pack Pinterest-style lunches (all while being well dressed while sipping our nonfat, half-sweetened, almond milk lattes). *Yah, okay!* The media and advertisements we are continuously bombarded with in our day-to-day life give an all-too-glamorized and terribly unrealistic portrayal of just how easy it's supposed to be. Suddenly being a mom and doing our best isn't good enough.

Did you know that the average American is exposed to more than three thousand advertisements a day? That's a whole lot of subliminal messaging thrown in our faces. We have become a society of women who preach support and female empowerment, yet we are riddled with unbridled external and internal judgments, comparisons, and crushing self-doubt. I always jokingly call Facebook and Instagram the *highlight reel.* We all do it, myself included. We love to show the great parts of our lives that we are proud of. The flowers our husband brings home *for no reason*, the perfect selfie while making cookies with our kids, the once-in-a-blue-moon self-care day. The problem is that we have no idea what is going on in this person's world. Maybe the husband brought home flowers because he forgot an anniversary. Maybe the mom who bakes fresh cookies works long hours and rarely gets time to do fun activities with her kids. We are so quick to post and share our victories and what we are proud of, yet we feel so ashamed to show the less perfect side, to keep it real and raw. It's far easier to hide this reality from the world. *Why do we assume life is always Disneyland for others? Why is it so scary to admit we are less than perfect (which is totally okay by the way!), to ask for help . . . to be vulnerable . . . to be real? Don't we all have things we aren't particularly proud of?*

As a result of self-comparison and doubt among other factors, both depression and anxiety in mothers are a greater epidemic than ever before. As mothers, we have adopted this external expectation of ourselves to conceal and suppress our emotions, hiding them from everyone. That's what I did. No one on the outside (or my family) had any idea about the soul-sucking pain and darkness I was experiencing. When you are having a rough day and joke that you need it to be "wine o'clock" or bedtime, take a moment to reflect on what's really going on beneath these jokes and steady stream of rough days. What are you hiding and what do you feel the need to conceal from the world? I learned how to hide, hide what I didn't like—the shame, the guilt, and the ugliness. *We are all kind of good at this, aren't we?* We think it's easier to hide the not-so-great parts of ourselves, but it's exhausting and lonely. Who wants to share their shame? It's terrifying, isn't it? It's a scary thing to let people in because we are forced to acknowledge and accept our own imperfections and insecurities. But I want to tell you it's okay to release those unjustified thoughts and negative self-talk. What would you tell your daughter if she felt that way? Now look in the mirror, Mama, and say the same thing to yourself . . . release it . . . release yourself.

Even as I sit here writing these very words, I'm filled with insecurities and self-doubt, feeling unworthy and imperfect. *Will this resonate with you, Mamas?* At thirty-seven years old I have three little girls who are counting on me to help them navigate the sometimes cruel world of womanhood. And FYI, I'm not always totally sure exactly how the hell I'm going to do that! Finally, at my age, I have discovered it is only when we are able to allow ourselves to be vulnerable with others that we are able to free ourselves from our shame and realize we are all alike in many ways. We are all connected in many ways, and our energy that helps create our mom tribe also dictates our mindset. When we feel overwhelmed and frustrated and are too focused on the stress of it all, we fall deeper into that negative thought cycle. The way we feel and *where* we choose to focus our attention and energy becomes an unconscious pattern. When we choose to focus on the positive and joy-filled parts of our day (even drinking a semi-warm cup of tea in the morning), we naturally shift our energy and notice more of the blessings all around us. And they are there . . . every day and everywhere, and when we take notice, they wrap us up in a warm, comforting, happy blanket. Mindset and energy shifts can be simple yet so impactful. Something as simple as reframing how we speak to ourselves can shift our entire mood. Any time you hear yourself saying "I have to," try saying "I get to." With that simple change in dialogue, you will no doubt feel more motivated and grateful. I would love for you mamas to explore self-love as some of the other amazing authors have written about. Mindfulness and self-love can be as simple as allowing yourself the time to sit and do nothing or whatever you want, free of judgment of yourself when you "should be doing something else." Letting go of the judgment is practicing self-love and self-compassion. When that negative self-talk rears its ugly head and freezes you dead in your tracks, think for a moment what you would say to your daughter if she were saying those very things to herself. Show yourself the same compassion and understanding . . . release those feelings.

Through my suicidal days and miscarriages, as well as almost losing my middle daughter, I found great inner strength. However, what I have come to realize and appreciate is that a woman's true strength is shown in the trials we face every single day. Our strength, *your* strength, shines through in how you show up in your life every day. Being a mom doesn't make us stronger, it shows us how strong we have been all along . . . maybe we just didn't know it yet. Sometimes motherhood, even as unbelievably fulfilling and purposeful as it is, can dim the light inside. The title "Mom" overshadows the woman underneath. I want to remind you that you are still there, even if you feel like you've lost a part of yourself, your identity, your abilities, your independence, or your individualism. I think many of us feel this way at some point, and we are not alone in those feelings. Here's the funny thing about these feelings: every other mom has felt the same thing. There are only so many feelings a person can experience, so no matter what season of life or motherhood you may be in right now, rest assured there is a tribe of mamas in this book who completely get it. Think about that for a moment and let it fill your heart with a calm sense of belonging. We really aren't as alone as we often feel. *Where* these feelings stem from and *what* triggers them will differ from person to person, but what you are feeling in this very moment is exactly what unites us all. We are not alone in this #momlife. We are doing the best we can, and I want to tell you that it *is* enough. *You* are enough. I love the saying, "Our kids do not need a perfect mom, they need a happy one," and I promise you, in their little eyes, *you* are perfection.

I know there is a sweet life to be lived through all the craziness and uncertainty that motherhood brings. Let's be honest: Our mental health takes a huge hit as a mom, no matter who you are or where you're from. I was so inspired and felt immense gratitude when I started openly sharing my journey with other mamas and had others share their stories and struggles with me. *That* is when I decided that my purpose was to help and serve others. I'd like to leave you with five takeaways that, if practiced regularly, can have a drastic and positive impact on your health and allow you to show up in your life as your best self:

Nutrition makes all the difference!

- Up to 95 percent of our serotonin production happens in our gastrointestinal tract, so what we eat directly impacts our mood and brain function.[6]
- Use simple tools like meal planners and shopping lists.
- Online grocery ordering services will be your best friend and saving grace.
- Use high quality and certified whole-food-based nutritional support supplements to bridge the gaps, including a clean, vegan omega blend.
- Shakes and pre-made breakfasts and snacks are fast and healthy options on the go (there are tons of ready-to-order services available, or Pinterest has some delicious healthy recipes!).

Move your body!

- Exercise releases endorphins that make us feel happy so basically move only on the days you actually want to feel better.[7]
- Go for a walk (most communities have mom fitness and/or walking groups).
- If on a time or budget crunch, YouTube or online at-home workout options are your BFF.

- Hire a trainer or join a gym.
- HIIT, Tabata, and interval training will show great results in a short amount of time, and no, you do *not* need to spend hours at the gym (unless that's your thing).

Be Mindful & Meditate!

- Practicing mindfulness (or even a few minutes of meditation a day) has powerful physiological impacts on our bodies.
- Use apps such as Insight Timer, Calm, or Headspace. YouTube also has great meditation music.
- Whenever you feel stressed or overwhelmed, stop and take five long, deep breaths (counting to five on the inhale and exhale).

Personal Development and Show Gratitude!

- What are you grateful for?
- Audible is a great audiobook app where you can plug into some great personal development audiobooks!
- Join a book club in person or online.
- Gratitude journals are a fantastic way to help us develop the habit of gratitude. I love the Five-Minute Journal.

Reach Out for Support!

- There are so many incredible resources out there whether you are suffering from postpartum depression, any type of anxiety, or just not quite feeling like yourself. Everyone needs some love, care, and a hand up from time to time as the demands of motherhood can be overwhelming.

- Ask your doctor for a referral to a counselor or psychologist.
- Use any medical/health benefits or employee assistance programs available for counseling or therapy.
- Ask family or friends for help when you need it—and do so unapologetically.

It has become my mission to help educate, motivate, and empower women to openly and unapologetically share their struggles while guiding them through their journey of rediscovering and redefining themselves as a woman beyond the title "Mom." I believe it truly takes a village, so let's make our village a strong, healthy, and powerful one. My wish for each of you incredible moms is to share your story because it matters, it's important, and it will inspire others. What would life look like if you let go of the shame, the guilt, the feelings of unworthiness and inadequacy? How would it feel to just release it all? How would your life change if you took just one small step toward feeling better? How would you show up differently in your life? Truly take a few moments to envision that. If ever you feel like your load is too much to bear, your heart is too heavy, your days and nights are endless, or like you just need a break, give yourself some much-deserved grace. Decide to treat your body and your being like the goddess you are because **you** deserve to feel good again. You are worthy, beautiful, strong, empowered, and un*bloody*stoppable! Be kind to yourself. Know that even if you feel like you've lost a bit of your spark or who you were, it is never too late to find yourself again. You WILL rise from the depth of the murky and sometimes suffocating water below and blossom into the beautiful lotus flower you are destined to be . . . that you already are. Above all, rest assured that **you've got this, Mama!**

It has taken time and a whole lot of false starts, good starts, and restarts.

– Christina Whelan Chabot
@mattersofmovement

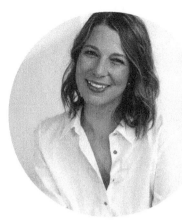

Christina Whelan Chabot

Christina's interest in health and wellness has been a lifelong commitment going back as far as her sixth-grade speech about health. She completed her undergraduate degree in physical education and health and her master's degree in the exercise sciences at the University of Toronto where she examined the positive impact of exercise on the nervous system. After graduation, although Christina was employed outside of her field of exercise, she continued to pursue her study of the human body through Pilates. She learned through Julia Wyncoll, the owner of Inhabit Pilates and Movement, Rucsandra Mitrea, the owner of Vital Directives, and last but not least, Dianne Miller and Mairin Wilde with whom she did most of her learning. Being the eternal student, she also began training as a Franklin Method™ educator with *the* Eric Franklin.

Christina has been teaching Pilates since 2008 and has worked with people from all walks of life. After having experienced the transformative process of having children, she was drawn to add a specialty in pregnancy and the postpartum phase so that she could *pay it forward* and share the help she was lovingly provided during and after her challenging pregnancies. A woman of multiple capes, Christina balances motherhood and a managerial position in her family's business along with Matters of Movement, a Pilates-based instructional practice she founded in 2017 so she could empower and connect with people, problem solve, and help them work toward the freedom that a fit and healthy body and mind will give them.

 mattersofmovement.ca

mattersofmovement

@mattersofmovement

~ To my beautiful family: Ray, Lucie, Norah, Austin, Carol, Richard, and Lina, and the amazing people in my village who have all held me up in one way or another.

Twelve

I AM MY NERVOUS SYSTEM
Christina Whelan Chabot

"Above all, be the heroine of your life, not the victim."

~Nora Ephron

WARNING*: This first part may trigger feelings of anxiety.*

Here we go again. The weight on my chest is making it hard to breathe. All I want is to catch my breath. To stop heaving. To get rid of this dead weight that keeps pounding on my chest. I'm trying to catch my breath, up and down, in and out, up and down, in and out. I'm okay. It's okay. It has to be, right? I feel like I'm inside a metal container as the sound of my pounding heart fills my ears and echoes all around me.

The sound around me is different, it's almost muffled.

I feel different. Detached even. Like I am not in my body.

I'm sweaty and tingly. It's not good. Oh, it's so not good.

The kids continue yelling because I'm not answering, and the baby feels heavy in my arms. I sit to gather my bearings, yet I feel so scattered and torn apart. I am so distracted by how I feel. My mind is swinging wildly—like a pendulum that shows no signs of stopping—from my body, to the sound of the kids, and back again. I can feel the panic setting in. If only I could retreat to something, anything, to make this go away. Somehow I manage to hear, *you've got this . . . it's okay . . . it'll pass . . .* so that I am able to get kid A set up for homework and get kid B a drink, but I'm a walking zombie while I simultaneously breastfeed kid C. *I have no clue how I'm functioning right now.* All I know is that I have no other choice.

Incidents like this one aren't precipitated by anything stressful. They just happen. One minute everything is completely fine, another, a case of sheer terror and panic—it's a slippery slope. Sometimes I'm sliding down this slippery slope because I realize that I can't find the health cards just as we're leaving the house to go see the doctor. *Darn it, where are they?!* I tear the house apart as I run through all the possible scenarios I will face when I show up without them.

On a good day, I fluctuate between calmness and low-level anxiety, which is where I most often find myself. I am not my best here. But I think of it as a location and not a state of being. This way I won't feel obligated to stay here. *I can leave at any time. Right?* That is the idea, anyway. Most people wouldn't stay at a party they weren't having fun at, right? *So, why am I always here? Ack!*

It is not just about the panic attacks and anxiety, it's the guilt. *Why am I not okay? We aren't struggling, we have good food, a stable home, a lovely community of family and friends, and so much to be grateful for. So, why this? Shouldn't I feel happy? Afterall, everything seems picture-perfect on the surface.* I don't feel entitled to these feelings. Yes, I parent alone most days and nights while my husband runs the family business, but I think of our moms who were often alone caring for us with little to no help.

What is it about me that is failing here? The guilt eats away at me, gnawing away at every fiber of my being, and it's hard to focus on anything else.

Like a lot of moms, I take on a lot. For example, I am still working a bit while on maternity leave, and I actively sought out to contribute to this book. Because, you know, I don't have anything else to do. But a calling is a calling. In a way, I'm still that little girl who fears missing out: compromising myself a little every time I say yes to something yet always wanting to feel relevant, capable, independent, and worthy.

❧

I know that some part of this is because of my fluctuating hormones. At three months postpartum, I rescue handfuls of hair from the drain after my shower. I am sleep deprived, I'm not eating well, and I seem to be needing a beer too often. Now you may wonder, *why doesn't she go to the doctor?* I did. I was referred to a great local mental health program for women in their first year postpartum. During my appointment, I was interviewed and all my answers to the more debilitating symptoms of postpartum depression were an emphatic *no*. Wanting to be clear about what I was experiencing, I added that I was having panic attacks, generalized anxiety, issues with anger and being over-touched, and a low libido. I could feel her prickle and cringe as I mentioned that last item. I almost laughed. *Why am I here if I can't talk about this?! Sheesh!* Looking back, I can see she was trying to triage the situation, but since I wasn't emergent, I could feel her interest in me waning. So I pushed even further and asked, "Am I a good fit?" In response, she offhandedly said if I didn't want medication, we could meet again and investigate talk therapy. With my emotions swirling around me like a swarm of bees, I left, feeling a mix of deep empathy for women experiencing symptoms worse than mine and as though I was falling through the cracks. I didn't go back.

So I'm on my own. It has taken time, some patience (which is in short supply), some self-forgiveness (also in short supply), and a whole lot of false starts, good starts, and restarts. Thankfully, I have a lot of tools under my belt, I just had to dig deep to piece them together.

Understanding the Autonomic Nervous System

I know this information may seem like a lot, but bear with me. The autonomic nervous system controls involuntary body functions and has two branches: sympathetic and parasympathetic nervous systems. The sympathetic nervous system (SNS) is known as the fight or flight response—the activator in times of stress that causes rapid breathing, heart rate, and sweating.[1] Although useful in situations of real and perceived danger, you don't want to function in that manner for prolonged periods of time. Sustained SNS activation through chronic stress has been linked to all kinds of health problems, such as anxiety, depression, high blood pressure, and addiction.[1]

Its counterpart, the parasympathetic nervous system (PNS), is your calming branch, the part that allows you to rest and digest. Ideally, you need a nice balance between the two branches. The way researchers assess this balance is through heart rate variability (HRV). When the SNS plays a greater role, like during times of stress, the time difference between each heartbeat is consistent, showing little variability. You'd think this would be a good thing, but it's linked to coronary artery disease, high blood pressure, and heart attacks.[2] When the PNS is actively working to balance out the SNS, the time between each heartbeat varies more, which is better for overall health.[3]

If you are like me, your body may enthusiastically lean on the SNS, jumping into action when a more subdued response is due. When this happens, I can't think clearly or concentrate. I don't connect with people and forget about accessing the parenting and coping skills I have so diligently armed myself with.

The prefrontal cortex is the part of the brain that controls our thoughts, decisions, actions, and emotions, all of which can be impaired by stress.[4] During unpleasant emotional stimuli, like when my kids are nearly tearing each other's eyes out in the back seat, the frontal activation is linked to higher heart rate or blood pressure, suggesting SNS activation.[5][6] So, when my SNS is overly active, it's no wonder that all rational thinking is out the window and all my trusty tools go to waste. It's also easy to see that we set ourselves up for failure every time we think we'll be able to whip out that amazing coping strategy when the going gets tough. It becomes a vicious circle.

What can we do? If you are like me, you might Google a thing or two (total eye roll here). But it's hard to sift through all the information out there. Coincidentally, while my PNS was active during a few quiet moments, I was able to see that my nervous system needed some love. I needed to reawaken my PNS so that the SNS could work in a real crisis.

Preventative Action

Prevention is easy to talk about and, at times, hard to put into action. Sometimes preventative methods are not clear, especially when we are too busy in reaction mode, so that we cannot access any preventative techniques. I want to share a quote from media moguls Cat and Nat (you may have heard of them):

> *I am the most perfect mom . . . when my kids are asleep, on a play day, generally out of the house or getting along perfectly. #momtruths*

First, I laughed because it is SO true, but then I thought, *Why not use these perfect moments to boost the PNS?* Bolster the PNS in preparation for times when you might be triggered by fighting kids or their attitudes and uncooperativeness. Train the PNS to be steadfast in moments of stress. Treat it like a muscle so that your "muscle memory" can kick in when your mind can't. You'll rarely be successful at using your coping mechanisms when you can't think straight, but I can tell you, you'll have more success when you are calm and that prefrontal cortex isn't being taken out of service by the SNS and stress hormones.

Exercise to Boost PNS

We all know exercise is good for us and the guilt is real when we think we can do more. Engaging in regular exercise improves the balance between the SNS and PNS. People who exercise regularly have a greater HRV than those who do not exercise at all,[7] giving them a protective health effect. Now, in looking at mental health, people with depression have shown less HRV.[8] Regular exercise is recommended in both prevention[9] and treatment for mental health.[10]

We recently moved and lost a bunch of help, and now that I am drowning in my responsibilities and so much laundry, who has time for exercise? Well, I do, in between all the other little things. I call it my *In-Between Workout.* Right now I don't have time for an uninterrupted thirty-minute session of exercise, but if you do, go for it and savor it. Until I do, I will squeeze in some squats, take the stairs a little faster than usual, go for a walk with the kids, or have a dance party. I like to commit to ten to fifteen minutes, and this way, it feels doable. It's not easy, but I do my best, and I vow to reserve guilt for a time when I am not stretched so thin. Plus, when I know I'm investing in my PNS, it makes me happy.

Franklin Method to Boost PNS

The Franklin Method™ is like a breath of fresh air and always brings ease and calm to my body. It is a practice that combines many important elements; however, one key element is the imagery work. Imagery has been used by athletes to visualize a specific or generalized aspect of their performance before a competition, which people sometimes call "psyching up." It has been so effective that it is standard practice for athletes to use this technique for performance enhancement in high-level competitions.[11,12]

Eric Franklin, the founder of The Franklin Method™, brings a similar imagery technique to everyone. You learn to observe changes in your body before and after activity by *integrating movement and using anatomical and biomechanical knowledge, movement-related imagery and sensory cues, proprioception, self-talk, and self-touch.*[13] It essentially teaches the student that the mind is a powerful transformative tool.[14] I originally began using this method with movement and my body, but I quickly saw its value in boosting my PNS and self-calming strategies in stressful situations. Instead of psyching up, I've been *psyching down.*

When I feel panicky, I don't feel right in my body and I detach—a bit like my onesie is now only covering half of my body. So before I start reasoning with my mind, first I need to get back *into* my body. Imagine climbing back into that onesie. I do that by using the proprioceptive ball techniques taught in the Franklin Method™ where you bring awareness to your body and tune in to the sensations by using the ball to tap on any area you feel may need it, moving from gentle to vigorous, or I move my body (cue Franklin Method™ movement sequences, dance party, or impromptu squats) so that I can *feel* my body. At other times, when I am calm and know I am entering a potentially stressful and triggering situation like school pickup before a long drive, I use positive imagery beforehand. I picture myself handling everything like a champ, and I think of the words I will use and how I will use them.

Breath to Boost PNS

I know, everyone says to breathe, and you may or may not have bought in. If you haven't, the science is there to show that deep and slow breathing leads to better health outcomes, including a better balance of the PNS and SNS, meaning more HRV, [15] an improvement in attention, negative affect, stress,[16] anxiety, and depression.[17, 18] Good, right?

So the question remains, what kind of breathing are we talking about? You might get a lot of different advice, but essentially, you want to inhale a nice, deep, lung-filling breath without any restrictions from the belly or ribs. Then you want to follow up with an exhale that is longer than the inhale. There are no steadfast rules, but if you need something specific, try doubling the length of the exhale. For example, if you inhaled for a count of three, exhale for a count of six. The reason is that the vagus nerve, which is responsible for PNS activation, is regulated by breath, specifically the exhale. The exhale is where the "psych down" happens. Make it work for you. A deeper, slower breath (specifically, the exhale) means that there will be more oxygen transfer in the lungs, a slower heartbeat (more PNS and HRV)[19] and lower blood pressure.[20, 21] How can you say no to that? All I can say is that I consciously work on my breath a lot. I have to with three kids constantly keeping me on the go—mentally, emotionally, and physically.

Talk Therapy and Tapping into My Village

Reducing stress has brought me the most success. Before baby number three, I felt overwhelmed, angry, unhappy, and generally like a failure as a mom. I knew it was time for help and luckily found a social worker who was a great fit for me. I went in looking for answers. *How can I be less angry? How can I be a better mother? How can I not screw up my kids? Fix me!* We talked about my coping mechanisms and circumstances: working full time and carrying the weight of parenting alone while my husband works long hours. I didn't get the answers I expected, but I did learn to rediscover my voice, manage expectations, be empowered, and understand others' trauma, which was impacting me in ways I was unaware of. I learned that when I am pushed beyond my limits, I can't think clearly, and I either shut down emotionally or get angry. I walked out with the biggest message of all: *Perhaps I am not the biggest problem. Maybe, just maybe, I am okay (GASP!) and there is nothing fundamentally wrong with me. Instead of trying to fix myself, I need to fix my circumstances.* But what about the self-help train that I was on? It was barreling down the tracks and I couldn't get off.

So began the shift. First, to figure out what I needed. That, by far, was the hardest part. Like, *do I really need someone else to fold my laundry? No . . . but, then yes.* Then the inevitable question: *Do I really want someone else to fold my underwear?! No!* Let's just say that the need overcame the want in this situation. The realities of having help mean that people are going to be in your messy life. It feels hard to accept, but by the time our son was born, I had gotten over myself and found two part-time helpers. Between the girls and my amazing mother-in-law, I had help five days a week for a few hours a day. It was great and financially manageable. Everyone was happier because I was building our village.

I also have friends and family who offered to help, and guess what?! I didn't refuse. Normally, I would have wasted time worrying about imposing, but being accepting of their help brought us all closer. I felt good and they felt good. It was a win-win. People talk about "the village" and how it looks different today. I have a village, I just needed to reach in. There is absolutely no shame in asking for help, accepting help, and taking the time to help yourself.

I still have bad days because, unlike my anxiety, my path to healing is just that: a path. It's a road to travel and not a destination. A good friend once told me, "Guilt and shame are unproductive emotions." She was right. They are paralytic and hold you down. I know that in the good and in the bad I am merely a reflection of my nervous system. It is of me, but it does not define me. If I look back into that mirror, I know that guilt and shame have no place here. Hope does, though. When I've had a terrible day, and I haven't been successful at boosting my PNS by breathing, exercising, using imagery, or getting help, I try to end the night with a little forgiveness, gratitude, laughter, and the knowledge that there is always tomorrow.

So, Mama, I know that motherhood may sometimes feel endless, but see if you can find the space within you to treat yourself with gentleness and kindness so that you can bring yourself back to center, back to yourself. Just remember: Perfect moms are unicorns. They don't exist. Know that every moment is a passing one and that you have the power to change it in whatever way you find possible, whether it is with one deep breath or another way that works for you. When in doubt, reach into your village—no matter the form. Know that we've got you, we see you, and we feel you. Ultimately, we are you. So please know, **Mama, you've got this**; *that* I can assure you.

The time has come to stand tall in our brilliance and illuminate this world with light.

~ Jodi Decle
@jodi_transformationalcoach

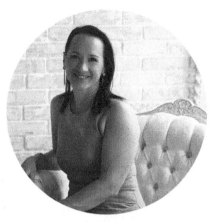

Jodi Decle

Jodi Decle is a deep, creative soul in love with life and the human spirit. She is a dedicated and loving mother to her three wonderful children and a transformational coach to women who are ready and committed to create the life of their dreams and step into their brilliance.

This empowering, inspirational woman knows through experience it is not only possible to transform yourself and your life by embodying your greatest self, but it is our greatest honor and investment. Having redesigned her lifestyle to align with her deepest values and highest mission, Jodi knows the transformation terrain inside out and helps her clients navigate this intuitively.

An advocate for mental, physical, and spiritual health, Jodi believes in taking full responsibility for what we truly want and bringing it to life through love, courage, empowerment, creativity, and joy. As a transformational coach, Jodi has had the pleasure of mentoring and supporting many women through their life-changing journeys.

She believes that being healthy goes beyond nutrition and exercise; being healthy invokes intuition and structure in service of flow, inspiration, creativity, and freedom. To her, health is a loving and honorable relationship between our body, mind, spirit, heart, and soul that works with our energy and emotions to keep us feeling grounded, nourished, balanced, strong, and alive.

You might catch her dancing, enjoying live music, running in nature with her husband, hiking to waterfalls, soaking up the sunshine at a beach, creating art with her children, or cooking up a fabulous dinner for her closest friends and family.

 jodidecle.com

jodideclecoach

@jodi_transformationalcoach

~ With deep gratitude to my longest-standing friend and example of a strong, resilient, and empowered woman: my mother, Esther. Thank you for being you, brilliantly and unapologetically. Thank you for always loving me and trusting me to find my own way. Because of your trust, I did.

Thirteen

EMPOWERED TO WELL-BEING AND BRILLIANCE
Jodi Decle

"Your job is to fill your own cup, so it overflows. Then you can serve others, joyfully, from your saucer."

~Lisa Nichols

There's a little girl who tells me she loves me "more than a million thousand unicorns, rainbows, and butterflies." She is sunlight for my spirit, and she lights up my heart. She is my Soleil Lucia Shalom, my five-year-old daughter who I prayed and longed for but wasn't sure I deserved.

Jaxen Phoenix is my loving and fiery middle boy—an eight year old with a madly creative spirit who is bursting with intense passion, inspiration, and humor. He counts on me to be a safe place for him to land and process his big emotions like frustration and anger as he navigates growing up in this world. My eldest sweetheart of a son, Isaiah Jason, at age twelve, has matured into a responsible, kind, and respectful young man who looks deep into my eyes and tells me he loves me and embraces me with his strong arms. He is both emotionally and intellectually intelligent, he loves learning, and he values close, meaningful relationships. I have come to know these three as my greatest gifts and teachers who indirectly show me where I still need to grow and evolve every day of my life. And when I think about making a contribution and having an impact through my own life, I realize that it begins most importantly in my own home by being a mother.

I see mothers as the most awe-inspiring, magical beings and feel simply amazed at what seems to be our capacity to *do it all*. With our strong intuition and deep devotion to love and nurture, we can be soft and strong, sensitive and resilient, hardworking, creative, and extremely resourceful. We are the mothers to the leaders who will carry this world into the future, and the time has come to stand tall in all our brilliance and illuminate this world with our light.

Isaiah's birth birthed me into a different person as old parts of me fell away and I stepped into motherhood. Although I became a mother instantly, twelve years later I am still balancing the *being* and the *becoming* of it all. Truth be told, I had a hard time adjusting to all the changes and extra responsibilities that swiftly came along. It felt like I had been living my life with training wheels on, only to wake up and find them removed altogether. Who knew the change from only having to be responsible for myself to now having a whole new human solely relying on me would throw me off balance?!

While trying to stay on top of everything and aiming to live up to the image of who my mother had been to me, I found myself feeling exhausted and overwhelmed. I was operating in a fog and running on empty. After all the to-dos were done to my standards, only then did I take a moment to think of myself and my needs, and by then my brain and body were fried, my energy: DEPLETED. Because of my lack of uninterrupted sleep, things like meal planning and self-care weren't done in a thoughtful, sustainable way (or at all). It was more like responding to emergency-like breakdowns. I pushed myself while running on empty. Even with my loving, supportive husband by my side being the amazing dad and partner that he is, I still allowed my own care and nourishment to always be an afterthought.

We had planned to have two or three kids (each separated by one or two years), but our learning curve with our firstborn made us reevaluate the rush to add another baby to the mix. Isaiah was four years old when Jaxen was born, and it felt good that we'd given ourselves that breathing room to grow into parenthood. Juggling our priorities, including my full-time career, had stretched me. I dreamed of my second maternity leave as if it were a year-long spa retreat.

To ensure both my baby boys got the love and attention they needed and deserved while still maintaining that spark and connection with my husband, I leaned into my feminine instincts and began trusting myself more as I naturally wove my love into them all. Still, I unconsciously fell back into the habit of only leaving myself crumbs for self-sustenance. The stress that I allowed in caused constant cortisol spikes, hormonal imbalances, and exhaustion once again, and I noticed my waist expanding. Years into being a mom, my belly was still so big that there wasn't much room left for my baby boys to sit on my lap and read stories. I was acutely aware that it was not a good indicator of health, and it deeply affected my self-esteem. I could literally feel myself hunching over, shrinking down, and hiding in the presence of others. I was so embarrassed by my body that I seemed to disown it and disconnect from it. On the outside, I was smiling and trying to forget about what was bothering me, but on the inside, my spirit was crying "save me." I pushed these feelings down and carried on.

Our baby girl, Soleil, was born three years after Jaxen, and she gave our family the feeling of deep fulfillment and completion. When she was less than a few weeks old, I began experiencing debilitating pain from muscle spasms in my neck and back. It killed me to not be able to hold or even feed her, and I had to move into my parents' home and rely on my mother's full care while my husband was at work. I was being treated with chiropractic therapy, and my chiropractor sternly warned me that I was putting too much pressure on myself to have everything perfect in my life and that I was not taking care of myself enough. He said this pain was just the tip of the iceberg, and if I wasn't careful, I could damage my body for life. There would be no going back.

Although this breakdown gave way to a mini breakthrough, and I did open up to receiving a little more support, my own stubborn desire to be fully self-sufficient and my resistance to asking for help or leaning on anyone closed off opportunities for friends and family to feel closely connected to me. Five years later, I am still working at it. "How do women do it all?" I asked myself then as I embarked on a mission to uncover the answers. I began interviewing mothers I admired and collecting insight. It was only years later that I realized the underlying belief hidden within my question was, in fact, the root cause of my recurring stress and exhaustion. I guess I hadn't fully heard and accepted the message from that chiropractor. I had to realize it again and again until it became my own truth and belief that we don't have to do it all!

The years of motherhood went by, and my spiral of learning and growing came in cycles: many more breakdowns, many more break-throughs. I would notice that pattern of depletion as I got swallowed up by responsibilities and stress. I kept pushing myself to do all the "doing," thinking I was fulfilling my vision of being a good mother. But when I took a closer look, my children weren't getting to see me and experience me in my joy, in my full radiance, in my creativity and light.

I had known for years the feeling of serving from an empty cup. It felt like tension and stress. I was holding it all together until it broke down and blew up, often through exhaustion and outbursts of anger and constant impatience followed by remorse and sadness. That was not me being my best and honoring my life. That was not who I really was and not the woman or the mother I was born to be. I knew there was more to me.

As a young girl, I was deep and sensitive but also deeply insecure. I strived to reach the top of my mother's high expectations and standards and looked to others for validation, acceptance, and approval. I can see her . . . the little girl who dreamed of being a dancer, who climbed trees and hung upside down from their branches, laughing and being silly, the one who disappeared into nature and sang from her soul all alone, stopping to breathe in the beauty of flowers and smiling at the trees when the leaves waved to her. The one who noticed the magic that the sun shone onto the ocean as it glimmered and sparkled . . . the one who always looked for deeper meaning and felt heightened emotions. The one who looked to the older ones from underneath her metaphorical deep waters of emotion that she was drowning in and screamed "save me." She is the precious little one who needed a hero to assure her that she is safe to be her beautiful, unique self in every color that her heart and spirit inspires her to be; that she is a gift not to be hidden, but to be brilliant for all to see.

For almost forty years, I lived not knowing my true potential for health and well-being. In and out of states of depression and self-loathing, I was unaware that I had been my own jail keeper, holding the key to my freedom all along—freedom away from an experience of victimhood and stress to a life of true health and highest service. One day, while sitting in a meditative state, I tuned in to a most beautiful vision of myself, freely and radiantly living my best life. There she was! My hero! She had let go of all that extra weight and healed from her past pain and trauma that it housed. She had become my very own savior and hero, and now that she had saved me, she was free to help others do the same for themselves. The feeling that washed over me as I saw Her and felt Her essence, completely lit me up. I fell in love with a feeling and a possibility of who I could be: my best self. I tuned in to my desire for this vision and I knew exactly why it was important to me on all levels. There was a fire burning in me like I had never felt before. Every cell in my body was vibrating with excitement!

That was the moment when everything within me aligned to make the biggest decision of my life: No longer could I, or would I, let the rest of my life go by and not experience what being Her was like. I decided to let go of everything that was holding me back, weighing me down, and keeping me stuck. I made the decision to believe in Her and love Her enough to bring Her to life!

I would bring Her to life to be an example for my children and for them to be mothered and loved by Her. I would bring Her to life so that others would know it was possible to have this kind of breakthrough to transform and to live their best lives too.

I was done with feeling insecure and unworthy. I was done with living in my head, chastising myself and constantly feeding myself shame, guilt, or fear. I was done with disowning my body, not feeling comfortable and at ease in my own skin, not feeling like I belonged or that I was good enough. And I was sure as hell done with unconsciously checking out and sabotaging myself. I knew I needed to get over *all those fears and limitations* if I was to be an example and serve others in the way that I desired. The instant that powerful decision was made, the rules of my world shattered. There was a massive demolition of old beliefs, limitations, and habits that came crumbling down in one shot as I made space in the realm of possibility for who I had decided to become. Like a refugee, I fled the caged existence of fear, victimhood, and regret and crossed the bridge of faith, empowerment, and forgiveness as I began to trust myself and love my vision into life. It started with a massive letting go of everything I was not . . . and it continued with an intense commitment of self-love and self-respect. I could feel the energy of excitement rising as other supportive decisions formed and took shape:

- A decision and commitment to live a life of true health and well-being
- A promise to my spirit to experience exercise as a fun and joy-filled activity, by choice and through mindset
- A promise to my body to respect it and nourish it with nutritious and delicious food (that would also fuel my brain), and let go of my unnecessary body weight
- The decision to be my own best friend and to commit to self-care
- The decision to hold onto my vision and trust the process by showing up and doing the work even when it was uncomfortable or scary

I knew the time had come to move with the energy of that excitement, paddle out to that massive wave of inspiration, jump on board and surf that wave like it was God's gift to me. I took massive action immediately by hiring a personal trainer, Nelson, and changing the way I nourished and fed my mind, body, and spirit for good.

I had to believe in myself enough to hold the vision with relentless conviction. I built an honorable and loving relationship with myself by keeping my word with every intention. I had to show myself I meant business. I designed my lifestyle to fulfill my vision and stepped into it day after day. Step by step, plank by plank, I created the structure I needed to feel *on track* with routines and check-ins and also gave myself the space to flow with my intuition and inspiration.

I very quickly fell in love with the joy, balance, and freedom I found in my new life. And the falling in love flowed into all the actions that supported my change and transformation. I fell deeper in love with learning about nutrition and being creative in the kitchen. I fell in love with the feeling of building my physical strength and endurance and the satisfaction of achieving things that were hard and that I never dreamed I could do.

One year later, when I did a professional photo shoot for my coaching business, it was clear to the outside world I had completely transformed my body. I was not only fifty pounds lighter, but I was also strong, fit, confident, and comfortable in my body for the first time as an adult. However, the more powerful and fundamental transformation had happened on the inside.

Along the path, my awareness amplified, and I faced and processed deep pain, disappointment, and many old stories, triggers, and emotions. It was hard as hell at times. I remember my husband finding me crumbled in anguish on the bathroom floor after a phone call with a loved one and another time running on the trails with tears streaming down my face.

My awareness gave rise to an embodiment of compassion, understanding, and forgiveness. I learned to hold my vision, despite any temporary conflicting evidence, and to gather even the smallest signs of my vision coming to life while celebrating every single milestone with gratitude and excitement. Space was created for healthy boundaries and growth. I leaned intensely on God's love and guidance, finding a way to use the pain as fuel to rise like a phoenix from the ashes of my old self. My relationship with God and trust in the unseen support became the hidden treasure of my transformation.

In my life now, "healthy" means a state of balance and flow between my mind, body, soul, and spirit. It means I have a trusting and respectful relationship with my whole self. It means being whole and present with my children (having taken care of myself so that I am showing up rested, resilient, fulfilled, and strong). I am intentional with my thoughts and my energy, honoring my inspiration, intuition, and emotion. Being healthy means being clear on who I really am and what I stand for. It means knowing what my priorities are and taking full responsibility for them. It is my journey and my practice of holding a vision, setting intentions, and co-creating. I have stopped showing up empty and relying on other people or things to fill me up. I take care of myself and love myself fully now. I have created powerful practices and habits that include gratitude, meditation, creativity, and visualization—all of which deeply nourish and restore my soul.

I have continuously and passionately educated myself about nutrition, and I delight in creating a menu of mouth-watering, delicious, and wonderfully healthy homemade dishes that we prepare as a family with the seasonal changes and on rotation. After working with an amazing personal trainer for one year, I now train regularly with my husband, Shawn, as my workout partner. I also do yoga and Zumba classes on my own. I went from hiding in the back row at my Zumba class to bravely inching my way up to the second row. I am now in the first row right beside my absolutely amazing instructor, Shelley (even though I am far from doing all of the moves perfectly). I cannot begin to describe the incredible joy and elation I feel as I dance (and I get to do it two to three times a week). I'd like to think that the little girl inside of me who dreamed of being a dancer dances with me every time. Sometimes, as I catch myself in the mirror beaming with the biggest smile on my face in the middle of our choreography, or I catch a glimpse of my body moving to the rhythm of the music and see new muscle definition that's taking shape, I silently connect in deep recognition of the present moment and the journey that has brought me here.

My husband, Shawn, also became my personal running coach and has been by my side every step of the way as I went from believing and experiencing that I could not run for more than five minutes without my chest burning and feeling out of breath and dizzy to becoming an avid runner and doing 5K races regularly. I humbly completed my first 5K in forty-four minutes (feeling on top of the world and celebrating with great emotion at achieving this time), then a little over a year later, I shocked myself with a twenty-seven minute new personal record. I remember the feeling as I ran past the finish line: My body fell to the ground as a tsunami of emotion released like a wave through me, and I had tears streaming down my face in gratitude to myself.

I have continued to minimize stress within our family life by keeping our priorities clear and simplifying and putting systems in place. These practices have instilled responsibility and time management while easing chaos and confusion. We now have a Sunday routine to set us up for a successful week ahead. Each of my children also have their own morning routines and simple weekly practices to ensure they are putting important things first.

My children love having my full presence, creativity, and magic in their lives. They have embraced all the simple structures that my husband and I have placed in our family life, which now enable us to thrive and be happy. Together we have lightened up with more play and are each growing into our best selves. It took consistent dedication and practice, but we are on the other side of that river of change now, and I can tell you that it was ALL worth it, and you can do it too.

I have discovered that we are the only ones who truly know who *we* are born to be and what we most deeply desire. We have the ability, and I believe, the responsibility to create our own fulfillment. Through my transformation, I can tell you that my best self truly came to life through my best health—living a healthy life (mind, body, spirit, heart, and soul). Not only am I being the best mother to my three beautiful children but I am also shining my light in service now. I stand for you and all women—to bring forth your own strength, wisdom, intuition, God-given beauty (inside and out), and to make your mark on this world. You are needed, Mama. You matter, immensely. I hope you empower yourself to fill your own cup and serve in the way that your heart and spirit calls you to, brilliantly. **Be your brilliant self, beautiful Mama!**

Section Three

SPIRIT

Featuring
Danielle Williams

Justine Dowd

Maria Blackley

Shayroz Khosla

Leisha Laird

OPENING COMMENTARY BY
Sabrina Greer

The *spirit* is often referred to as the nonphysical part of a person that is the seat of emotions and character, also known as *the soul*.[1] In religion and philosophy, the *soul* is the immaterial aspect or essence of a human being and is considered synonymous with the mind or *thy self*. In theology, the soul is further defined as that part of the individual that partakes of divinity and sometimes thought to survive the death of the physical body.

If you would have told me a few years ago that *spirituality* was connected to either *health* or *motherhood*, I would have laughed out loud. I would have told you to spare me and leave it for the Sunday School kids. Don't get me wrong. I have nothing against organized religion or church and have always had a very **you do you** outlook on the whole thing. As a child to a Catholic mother and an atheist father, neither practicing much of anything, I always related church to boring weddings and sad funerals. It wasn't until I started traveling that I discovered my god—the Universe, Source, Higher Power; call it what you will. I had always thought of spirituality outside of organized religion as a tad nonsensical. When I went to university, I studied old school psychology, you know, structuralism and introspection, the study of thoughts and the mind as science. The idea that *essence* or a wisp of stardust existed within us was beyond my amateur arrogance.

I think it was actually on my trip to Cusco, Peru, six years ago when my narrow mind cracked wide open to the possibilities of the divine and my spiritual journey began. It was day three of a six-day hike through the Andes on a remote path alongside the Inca Trail. The altitude was high (higher than I had ever experienced), and the weather was expectant for that region in January (everything from twenty-five degrees and sun, to minus five and snow). I have never seen such a pendulum. I had been pushing mental and physical limits I didn't even know I had or that were possible. I was past the point of *no return* (something 40 percent of the participants did when they had the chance on day two—return home), but I was on a mission to prove something to myself. A few months prior to this journey I had endured a heart- and ego-crushing breakup, and I had a nonrefundable ticket to anywhere Peruvian Airlines flew. We had booked a trip with a bunch of couples for *him* to supposedly propose marriage to me atop a mountain with alpacas and snowcaps. I guess he lost the memo somewhere that you shouldn't marry someone when you are having a long-term affair with someone else, but we will save that story for another book too.

That night, three thousand meters above the world I knew, after thirteen straight, grueling hours of hiking terrain like no other on this planet, we set up camp in the most beautiful, mountainous, and pic-turesque vision I have ever seen. I silently wept. If you know me, this is unusual. There were multiple rainbows, like seven, and rays of light hitting the rolling green ridges and snow-covered peaks, wildflowers, and mountain goats. It was an Impressionist painter's dream. Breathtaking was an understatement. Our porters and chefs had set camp already and prepared a delicious meal of Cuy (I will let you Google that one but wouldn't if you are vegan) and quinoa soup. After we stuffed our tummies, it was time for bed. Our tents were small and uncomfortable. I had had a hard time relaxing the previous few nights and had only passed out from sheer exhaustion. That night was different, though.

That night I fell into such a meditative state; that night I saw God. I had started studying the art of meditation on the airplane to Peru, twenty-three days before this experience, and I had been attempting to calm my mind without distraction for many months before that. There, in the beauty of the Andes, heartbroken, emotionally lost, thinking this was it for me and this life, knowing if this hike didn't kill me, the reality of heading home to the absence of my house, my partner, and my career would certainly do the trick. There, mountainside, in the pouring rain, in a tiny little tent, I did it. I finally quieted my mind. We are talking third-eye, out-of-body meditation, clarity of the purest kind. This was the moment I knew there was more to us than our physical bodies and consciousness, that we were part of a bigger cosmos. I felt the Universe's power and unconditional love come over me like a tsunami of warmth.

After that trip, I became a student of the Universe. I read every book, went on meditation retreats, and started a spiritual practice (because let me tell you, it is practice). I realized that a major piece of my overall health and wellness was this practice; it was the missing piece to my puzzle. My physical and mental health were sound, but my spiritual health was missing. I realized that spirituality is synonymous with hope, belief, and fate, and it is what gives us the strength to move forward, regardless of how impossible it may seem.

In this section, you will meet the warriors who applied their version of this practice to help them through their difficult times. We discuss *surrendering* to the greater plan and holding space for *forgiveness*. Spiritual health may be the most difficult of the three to achieve. Human nature is to be skeptical and to believe in only what we can see. To be truly healthy, however, we need to live a holistic life and be sound in body, mind, *and* spirit. This is what makes us whole.

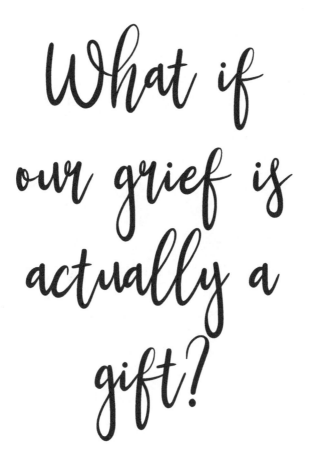

What if
our grief is
actually a
gift?

~Danielle Williams
@danielle.g.w

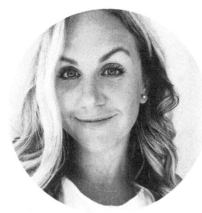

Danielle Williams

Danielle Williams had an idyllic childhood attributed to small towns, big dreams, and the best family in the world. From a young age, she put pen to paper and was the recipient of many young author awards. After university, Danielle began a career in personal finance, and made her best decision yet—she married the love of her life, Russ. Though she has traveled much of the world, her heart remains firmly planted in the foothills of Alberta, Canada.

After the loss of her firstborn, Roark, Danielle began writing more extensively, publishing her first in-print venture in the book, *You've Got This Mama, Too.* She is currently working on a lead author series for bereaved parents and is also a presenter and author on financial literacy topics. You can find her personal musings and writing on Instagram and her website.

Danielle is an entrepreneur at heart and an avid early riser, coffee drinker, and spirit junkie. She counts her lucky stars to be chosen to parent Sterling and Bronwen, and she holds her spirit babies, Roark and Ellie, in their ever-loving light. Danielle firmly believes in the philosophy that there are gifts in all trauma—our goal is to find them and then share them with the world.

daniellewilliams.com

@danielle.g.w

- For Russell, Sterling, Bronwen, Roark, and Ellie—my entire heart, infinitely. In our family, we share sorrow, and we share joy. And we always keep our chins up.

Fourteen

BREATHE. HOPE.
RISE. GODSPEED.
Danielle Williams

*I was lucky enough to have hit rock bottom
before, right? So I know, for a fact, that rock
bottom is always the beginning of the newness.
It hurts and is painful, and then there's the
waiting—where you don't know what the hell is
going on and you don't think any of it is going to
make sense and then—there's the rising.*

~Glennon Doyle

Heartbreak, Again

My midwife scans my belly for the heartbeat. Her brow is furrowed. I am
not worried. She is a student and the more experienced one is playing
with our daughter, Sterling, who is seven months old and babbling to
the midwife. She is playing pat-a-cake and Sterling is giggling. It makes
me smile. I am going to have two children within twelve months of each
other. Irish twins they sometimes call it, though I am not sure that's
politically correct anymore. Certainly, this baby was a surprise, though a

welcomed one. *Any parents who have lost a child will know what a miracle each baby is.*

The student stops and heaves a sigh of frustration. She asks for the more senior midwife, and they exchange positions. The student is now playing with Sterling. The more experienced midwife pushes around my womb, and the monitor is static—the whoop-whoop we are all straining to hear is completely nonexistent.

"Okay," she says. "Let's send you in for an ultrasound and double-check. I am sure everything is fine. You are ready for the anatomy scan anyway."

"Yes, it's booked for later this week," I reply.

"They can combine appointments," she says. "Today, though."

She helps me off the bed and makes the arrangements for her assistant to book me in. I gather my things and pick up Sterling, smelling her still-delicious baby smell, recalling the most relief I have ever felt—the moment I held her in my arms.

I call my husband, Russ, and tell him what has happened. He says he is on his way. In our first three pregnancies, he attended every midwife (and OB) appointment. Now he attends just the most pertinent ones. That sounds really cold, but really, it is a practicality that all multiple-loss parents understand. I drop Sterling off with a family member and drive to the Maternal-Fetal Medicine clinic. Maren Morris's "80s Mercedes" is playing on the radio as I pull in. I really like that song. And I know that I will never forget that moment.

❧

Russ is holding my hand. The jelly is warm and the wand is moved aggressively across my belly. The ultrasound tech is young, maybe twenty-five. She doesn't say anything. I am holding my breath. I have a sinking feeling that I know all too well. I feel light-headed and anxious, and then she finally says, "I am sorry. There is no heartbeat."

My breath escapes me. I am numb. Russ's head collapses into his hands and he is crying.

Again.

This has happened. Again.

I want to run: from my reality of our losses; from the pain that I know lies ahead of us.

Forty-four hours after her heartbeat wasn't detected—with inconceivable heartache—Russ held me up as I gave birth to our third child and our second daughter. A still baby girl. We named her Ellie Aurora. Aurora as a ROAR tribute to the first soul she ever met, her brother Roark.

And the night we returned home from the hospital, Aurora lights danced across Western Canada.

❦

A week or so later, I am rocking Sterling, and I am singing to her. My favorite lullaby. One that cuts right to my heart and connects me with all my children. It is "Godspeed (Sweet Dreams)" by the Dixie Chicks.

Sterling is so little and yet chronologically not the youngest of our children. I am still recovering from the birth of her sister. Gratitude and melancholy overcome me. I promise myself in that moment that I will always be satisfied with our family as is, that no matter what happens, my darling Sterling Sophie is enough. And I tell her that. And then I turn off the lamp and pull her close as we drift together.

Gratitude Summons Me

After we lost our premature son, Roark, I felt my life take a path which I now label Grief, Gratitude, Grace. I felt so many gifts of gratitude that led me to the grace of acceptance and hope in my grief journey. Roark wasn't our first loss. And I have heard it all.

"At least it was early." (Baby 1, miscarriage at 8 weeks.)

"At least you got to meet him and hold him." (Roark, born prematurely at 26 weeks.)

And now,

"At least you were not full term." (Ellie, born still at 19.5 weeks.)

At least, at least, at least. We live in a culture of comparison. And I have been told to classify Ellie as a miscarriage, not a stillbirth. I used to feel pained by that sentiment. Now I care much less about the classification. I birthed her. I was painfully induced for twenty-four hours until the contractions started. And on all fours, I pushed her out of my body. A moment of relief and escalation that was shadowed by the lifeless, tiny baby that came with it. And yet (and this feels so intimate to share), it was beautiful, filled with love and miracles. The sun was just rising, and in that moment, Russ and I cried in sadness and gratitude. It was a delivery I was told I would never have. *A vaginal delivery*, Russ holding and coaching me. After Roark's emergency classical cesarean section, I was told I would never labor for risk of uterine rupture. So Sterling was born via cesarean section, and Ellie was to be too. Only she was small, and the risk for rupture tiny. So I labored. Ellie's gift to us.

Ellie's gift (and my ability to receive it) transformed my grief and changed its shape and size again. *Life is filled with much ease when we focus on what we have rather than what we are missing.* It has taken me a long time to get here, though. Loss is not something that ever leaves. Yes, it changes;

however, it's a constant. I have learned that I can make things harder for myself, or I can find some peace—some gratitude in grief.

If someone said this to me before I was ready to see it, I might have closed the doors. I had a choice point: stay in the swamp of pain, revisiting it with the same eyes, thoughts, conversations with others, or—*rise*—shift my story and hold all my children in light and parent them in the unique way they have offered to be parented.

As bereaved souls, we must invite joy back into our lives. Slowly and steadily. Joy is all around us if we stay in the now and appreciate it. For me, it is simple things like hot coffee and the smell of fresh mornings and rubbing my dog's belly. It's the laughter of my daughter, picking berries on a warm summer day, or the goodwill of a stranger. And after I invited a bunch of *little joys* back in my life, I was able to feel the big joys—like excitement and hope for the future.

Collectively, to stop the joy drainage, we need to stop the comparison of birth stories and death stories and classification of loss. Loss is loss, and we all experience it differently. Each of my losses pained me. Roark was the catalyst for my life's direction and change. And yet his significance did not diminish the pain I felt in losing Ellie. After her death, I had to go easy on myself and take the healing steps again. Through my most tense days, I have learned that mental health needs to take priority as do spiritual health, and physical health, and well, health. *Vitamin P (pleasure) needs to be taken in daily.* Healing takes conscious effort. I like to think of our mind, body, and spirit work as the best and hardest work. It is the most rewarding, most challenging.

❧

About a year after Roark passed, my husband and I were invited to join a grief group. After much deliberation, we agreed to attend the first session to "see how it goes." After one hour of hearing the stories of ten other families, there was no turning back. We felt seen. We felt heard. We felt understood.

We were *not invisible* to this group.

And in the twelve weeks we spent together, I told our grief group that I would die if I lost another child. I actually said that out loud.

And yet, here I am.

Our connectedness to other grieving families helped us heal and walk *with our grief* rather than from it. Because hope is so powerful when it is shared between warriors.

Francis Weller, a grief therapist and renowned writer has said this: "The work of the mature person is to carry grief in one hand and gratitude in the other and to be stretched large by them. How much sorrow can I hold? That's how much gratitude I can give. If I carry only grief, I'll bend toward cynicism and despair. If I have only gratitude, I'll become saccharine and won't develop much compassion for other people's suffering. Grief keeps the heart fluid and soft, which helps make compassion possible."

On that note, he asks, "How many of us have ever been thankful for our grief before?"[1]

Woah. What if our grief is actually a gift?

This thought helped me immensely. If we eventually lose everything we love then we really need to learn how to walk with loss, even when our loss is as traumatic as a child's death. Even when our loss is multiplied—death after death after death. Even when we are hoping to expand our family again. Even when there is risk for more heartache.

Because we can be both hopeful (even joyful) and also grieving.

We can be healed—and still healing.

Surrender, Completely

For a long time, I (once again) was stuck and focused on why we lost another baby. *Hadn't we learned all we were supposed to after Roark? What purpose did the Universe have in store for us after losing another child? What kind of test was this? Did I fail the first one?*

Darkness.

I relied on the light-filled people around me to support me through the pain. I connected deeper with bereaved families. I was reminded that we don't get just one thing in life to struggle through. And no one is immune to suffering. There is so much varied suffering in this world, and we all suffer. I met "Why us?" with "Why not us?"

Still, growth is uncomfortable.

I had to surrender in total faith.

I know now that our story was prewritten. Believe me—I fully did not after Roark passed. I was angry at God and spiraled into all sorts of questions about life and my purpose here. Death is nothing short of utterly painful for the living. We are gutted. And yet my experience in holding Roark as he passed, and again when birthing our still baby girl, Ellie, was that passing and transitioning hold elevated moments that are beautiful and love-filled. Those moments helped me realize that death is only bliss for those that transition.

Even for our children.

It's hard to write that phrase because at some level it still feels totally unfair, even with the knowing that both of our spirit babies are totally okay and fulfilled and in bliss.

And I know there will be some who have lost children who won't agree with me. And that is totally okay. Because we all have our own journeys. I hold you close as you navigate yours. And I have completely surrendered in mine.

I am thinking about this all the time now. My journey and purpose. My spouse's journey and purpose. Our children's journey and purpose. As a mother, my only goal is to guide our children to fulfill their soul's purpose and journey.

Sterling knows about Roark and Ellie. She will forever be the girl sandwiched by angels—and how lucky for her to have so much love guiding her. The other night I walked into her room and she was sitting on her small toddler bed, Roark's lion in her arms. She was tracing his face and smiling. I asked her how she was feeling and she said, "Happy." She often asks me if I am okay, or if I am sad or happy. Her magnitude of feeling all emotions at two and a half years old is always a reminder of our capacity in life. And that is way more than we can imagine.

She reminds me to invite joy. Invite hope. Invite miracles.

Fast forward to February 2018—Russ and I are asked to chat on a radiothon in support of the Alberta Children's Hospital. So much of our healing is helped with walking through our grief rather than shouldering it. As Najwa Zebian so perfectly posed, "Those mountains you are carrying, you were meant to climb."[2]

The evening before the radiothon we had dinner with my sister and brother-in-law. We had a bit of wine and a lot of oysters and shellfish. I woke up in the night sick to my stomach. I couldn't hold anything in. I didn't know if it was food poisoning or nervousness about being live on the radio. In the morning, I asked the crew how they all felt/slept. I knew Russ had slept like a baby. Sure enough, everyone was well.

Little did I know that my sickness was another sign of a miracle. As we talked about our grief experience and the miracles that helped us through so much pain, a new, bold miracle was growing inside me.

Today as I write these words, my belly moves. It is growing, and our youngest daughter is kicking and rolling and showing me so much certainty. I have surrendered in total faith. *She will be healthy. She will be here to stay. I am healthy, and I am okay.* My faith mantra.

Being pregnant for the fifth time has been an awakening—never have I felt so guided outside of my being, and by love. Life is so full of big moments. All of them (especially birth and death) hold so much love. And grief feels like love I can't quite grasp. It always has me hoping for more. More signs, more memories, more earthly learnings and touch points with Roark and Ellie (and others I've lost).

Being pregnant after loss is not for the faint of heart. Long gone are the days of total naïvety and easy optimism. Each piece of pregnancy now holds a trigger week, a celebration or a pained memory, and So. Many. Tests.

So I focus on the miracle.

Albert Einstein said, "There are only two ways to live your life: as though nothing is a miracle or as though everything is a miracle."[3] There are signs of miracles all around us if you are open to them. And if you don't know what I mean, I am certain, one day, you will.

Because I have experienced the miracle of birth and the devastation of death, I have learned what a precious privilege it all is.

Because of *all* of our children, I have known the highest peaks and lowest valleys.

Because grief is forever and infinite, as is the possibility of love, hope, and joy.

And because I accept all of that, my life is full of gratitude and moments of grace.

I am a lucky one.

🪷

To all the parents in full bereavement who can't imagine a day fog free or filled with ease. I want to tell you that even though nothing can mend the cracks in your heart, within your brokenness is a uniqueness that when tapped into, is stunningly beautiful. Wounded healers are born. My wish for you is to turn your brokenness into empathy and move your new awareness toward a higher good. As a friend promised me, it will be energizing. Empathy to energy. Above all, I see you. You are not invisible. I pray you feel the army of love supporting you here, and from above. Hoping and believing in you to Rise Up. The Universe, and God, and the angels, and all of your fellow bereaved parents have your back.

If you take the
time to listen,
your heart
will tell you
what it needs.

- Justine Dowd
@justinedowd.phd

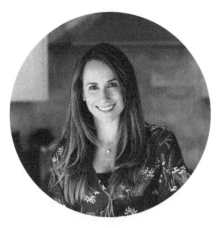

Justine Dowd

Compassionate, genuine, and insightful, Justine is passionate about empowering others to heal themselves holistically. A dedicated researcher, she has always been fascinated by the psychology of behavior change, which led her to complete a PhD in Health Psychology. Justine found an unexpected muse when she discovered that she had celiac disease immediately before she began her doctoral studies. The diagnosis would not only influence her lifestyle but shape her future. Justine focused her work on the dietary behaviors of people living with celiac disease, which earned her a number of research awards early on in her career.

Justine made the connection between life experience and professional passion again after both she and her husband struggled with "undiagnosed infertility" for over two years. During this time, Justine was inspired by the teachings of Kristen Neff and Brené Brown where she learned about self-compassion and found the courage to be vulnerable. After cultivating greater empathy for herself, Justine was motivated to help others do the same.

Justine's popular Gut Health Seminars and Holistic Fertility Retreats allow her to connect with kindred spirits. There, she shares her personal experiences, scientific knowledge, and loving support to help others find natural solutions for their gut health and fertility challenges. When she's not spending time with her family, Justine enjoys wine and soulful conversations with an amazing group of women she's blessed to call best friends. Justine lives in Calgary, Alberta, Canada, with her husband, two sons, and fur baby, Callie.

 justinedowd.com

justinedowd.phd

@justinedowd.phd

~ To my incredible husband, Lee: I wouldn't be where I am today without your unwavering love and support. Liam and Caleb: Thank you for choosing me to be your mama. You have brought more joy into my life than I ever could have imagined. To all of my supportive friends and health care providers who helped me get to the other side of the biggest mountain I have ever climbed: thank you from the bottom of my heart.

Fifteen

DARING TO HOPE: FINDING SELF-COMPASSION ON YOUR JOURNEY TO CONCEIVE
Justine Dowd

"A moment of self-compassion can change your entire day. A string of such moments can change the course of your life."
– Christopher K. Germer

Struggles with Fertility

What is wrong with me? I am young and healthy, married to the love of my life—why can't I just get pregnant? Such thoughts ran constantly through my head for over two years. Often overwhelmed by grief and anxiety, I would feel so frustrated. It seemed I had zero control over something that was so *easy* for so many people, and I would often find myself inconsolable. The seemingly smallest things would set me off: a friend being thoughtful and letting me know she was about to send out baby shower invites for a mutual friend or seeing a pregnant woman walking on the street. And then there were the bigger things: nonstop pregnancy announcements at girls' nights, on social media, and at work. I was so vulnerable that I would get triggered by the smallest of things, leaving me in tears for hours. I felt ashamed that I couldn't get pregnant. I felt frustrated that my body wasn't working as it *should*. I felt jealous of other women who just *became pregnant*. I felt like I wasn't *good enough*—not good enough as a wife or a woman. I constantly felt that I was letting down my husband and our families. It was awful.

I dreamed of becoming a mother since I was a little girl. At two and a half years old, I was ecstatic when little sister was born—my first baby! I loved being a big sister, and at six years old, when my brother was born, I became my mom's right-hand woman, jumping in to help with anything and everything I could. I loved being involved in diaper changes, feedings, and snuggles. My two-year-old stepsister came into my life several years later and made me an even happier big sister. Ever since then, I had this deep sense of longing for the day I would have my own baby. *My core ached to be fulfilled by becoming a mother. So why wasn't it happening for me?* I tried to stay as relaxed as possible, but after six months of trying with no luck (not even a single positive pregnancy test), I felt so lost, helpless, and anguished, thinking it might never happen for us. I wrote an entire chapter on this journey, and our ultimate answer, in my first co-authored book, *You've Got This, Mama, Too*

Coping with Infertility

So how did I cope? Well, it certainly was a roller coaster. However, the Universe was, and I believe always is, looking out for me—for all of us. As a part of my postdoctoral research, I happened to be studying the topic of **self-compassion**. I was learning all about how to practice self-compassion and the benefits of practicing it on a regular basis. As difficult as it was to be kind to myself during one of the hardest times of my life, the more I read about self-compassion, the more I knew I had to practice it to help me not only survive my fertility challenges but make the most of them and thrive on my journey with infertility.

What Is Self-Compassion?

Before I get into the formal definition of, and research on, self-compassion, I invite you to reflect for a moment on how you would treat a friend who was struggling or going through a difficult time if they came to you for advice or support. What sorts of things would you say to your friend? What tone of voice would you use? How would you try to make them feel? Take thirty seconds and write down or make a mental note of these things, particularly noting how you want to make your friend feel. I'm serious—actually stop for thirty seconds and reflect.

Now I invite you to reflect on how you typically treat yourself when you are struggling or going through a difficult time. What sorts of things do you say to yourself? What tone of voice do you use? How does it usually make you feel? Take another thirty seconds and write down or make a mental note of how you typically treat yourself when you are going through a difficult time. What similarities or differences do you notice between how you treat yourself and how you treat other people? Are you much kinder to other people than you are to yourself? Don't worry, you aren't alone. Research shows that 80 percent of people are kinder to others than they are to themselves, and almost no one treats themselves better than they do other people.[1] The problem is, when we are continually so hard on ourselves, it can make feelings of anxiety, depression, loneliness, and anger only get stronger, ultimately increasing the amount of suffering we endure during difficult times.[1] When I was dealing with infertility, I struggled most with feeling isolated—like I was the only person I knew who didn't have a baby. Having to go through numerous demoralizing tests and treatments, I honestly felt like an alien when I compared myself to other women who became pregnant so easily. One of the reasons I think I took infertility so hard is because I just expected pregnancy to happen quickly. I defended my PhD in June 2014 and expected to be well on my journey to motherhood soon after. For so long, my identity was as a student with a strong focus on academia, and that was all I knew. My core identity was challenged when I didn't transition from PhD Justine to Mama Jus. *Who am I now?* I felt so lost and anxious during that time, and these thoughts bubbled into self-doubt, self-deprecation, and of course, being unkind to myself on more than one occasion. These thoughts and behavior eventually led to more confusion, self-doubt, and a decrease in self-esteem—all because I thought my body simply hated me and didn't want to cooperate with me after everything I was putting it through: the fertility treatments, the tests, the multiple different diets, and of course, doing everything in my power to stay "relaxed" and have "fun." As much as I knew all the facts and how it could impact someone, I didn't think for a second that my self-worth would be so heavily impacted.

For decades, most psychological health research has been focused on boosting self-esteem to promote resiliency and optimize development. Today there are still numerous self-esteem-boosting programs delivered globally. Although the intent behind these programs is good, the fundamental issue with focusing on self-esteem falls in the definition of self-esteem itself. Self-esteem is one's evaluation of one's self-worth or value.[2] This definition inherently encourages *comparison* and *evaluation* of the self and of what others think of oneself, which may be one of the reasons why society is plagued by feelings of *not good enough*. Boosting self-esteem can be very difficult because it often entails encouraging people to adopt an unrealistic view of themselves.[1,3] Unfortunately, when our identity or sense of self-worth is challenged (i.e., we go through a difficult time in life), it doesn't always stand the test—people with high self-esteem are not more likely to effectively cope with the challenge than those with low self-esteem (see Neff[1] for a further discussion of self-esteem versus self-compassion).

I can relate to these research findings. Although I feel that I have a healthy level of self-esteem, it did nothing for me while I was struggling with infertility. If anything, I would often think, *I can do pretty much anything else that I set my mind to—why can't I do this? What is wrong with me? Why am I not good enough to become a mama?* Whenever I heard that someone else was pregnant, it felt like a direct attack on my self-worth and my identity, pushing me deeper and deeper into a dark hole of childless emptiness. I kept thinking to myself, *When will it be my turn*? I kept being hard on myself and my body, and it soon took a toll on certain relationships and friendships, which then crept into the various facets of my life. Such were the aftereffects of having my identity, my worth, my very essence as a woman questioned—*by society, my body, and mostly myself.* If self-esteem is the evaluation of one's worth and value, then self-compassion is at its core compassion, love, and kindness for oneself.

Self-compassion is associated with less judgment of oneself (and others), self-kindness, healthy behaviors, and protecting against the negative effects of self-criticism.[1] Fortunately, research over the past decade has shown that one can actually learn how to be self-compassionate. Self-compassion can be thought of as a "positive emotional stance toward oneself" and is defined as "giving ourselves the same loving kindness that we give other people."[1] I do my best to listen to my gut through meditation, and at this point, my gut told me that I was on a longer journey to motherhood than initially expected. I realized that I needed to work on my practice of self-compassion. I started with practicing regular meditation more frequently, adding in regular yoga classes and joining a year-long chakra journey. I figured, if I am going to get there on the Universe's timeline instead of my own, then I might as well learn how to start loving myself again, how to be kind to myself for a change, and then see what happens. And so it was. Thus, self-compassion does not involve any evaluation of the self. There are three main components of self-compassion: self-kindness, common humanity, and mindfulness.[1]

What do these three components actually entail? When we practice self-compassion, we are kind to ourselves rather than harshly self-critical. We recognize when negative thoughts go through our head and actively work to replace them with more positive ones (*self-kindness*). Negative thoughts played a key part for me when struggling with infertility. Thoughts such as *What is wrong with me?* and *Why can't I just get pregnant?* would swirl through my mind almost every second of every day. I was so hard on myself and felt so angry and frustrated at my body for not doing what I felt it was meant to do. The awful way I automatically spoke to myself was tough and made each month that passed more difficult. But through the initial pain of getting a negative pregnancy test or unwanted period, I would then begin with speaking kindly to myself, reminding myself that *I am loved and worthy of love even if I am not pregnant*. When experiencing infertility and going through the many challenges it brings, it can be easy to feel isolated and alone and as if no one has ever felt this way before. Practicing *common humanity* means we recognize that going through difficult times is a part of being human. Everyone struggles in their lives at some point in time. Try to remind yourself that you are not the only one who is struggling to conceive or going through multiple losses. Other women *have, are,* and *will* continue to go through it as well. This concept of common humanity is a key part of the mission behind the *You've Got This, Mama* community. We are here to let you know that *you are not alone.*

Finally, the third component is practicing *mindfulness* rather than over-identifying (or ruminating) over a situation. When we practice mindfulness, we acknowledge our feelings with non-judgment and acceptance. It can be easy to let trying to conceive (TTC) take over your life. I remember googling things I *never* thought I would type into my phone—all the crazy potential symptoms that might mean that this was finally my month. If you find yourself doing the same, it can be helpful to take a step back, take three deep breaths, and ask yourself: What do I need right now, in this very moment? Is it a warm bath? To call a friend who understands? To go for a walk in nature? If you take the time to listen, your heart will tell you what it needs, and this will help you cope with and process the emotions rather than allow you to spiral down the endless rabbit hole of abundant knowledge (known as Google) that can drive you bonkers.

Practicing Self-Compassion

When I was struggling to get pregnant, I would often think recurring thoughts including, *What is wrong with me? Why won't my stupid body just get pregnant? I must not be good enough to become a mother.* When you write it down and reflect on it, you can see how these thoughts are unlikely to be helpful when going through a difficult time. As I began practicing self-compassion, I began acknowledging when these thoughts would go through my head. I would then place my hands over my heart, take a deep breath, and say to myself: *Struggling with fertility is incredibly difficult. You are justified in feeling sad, mad, frustrated, and jealous. Try to remember that other people have felt this way too; millions of women all over the world have struggled with fertility issues as well. I'm here for you, I love you, and I don't want you to suffer.* This affirmation encompasses all three components—being kind to myself, common humanity, and being mindful. A shorter mantra that I often used was: *This is all part of MY journey; everyone has a different journey in life, and for some reason, fertility struggles are part of mine.*

Putting your hands over your heart can also be a very powerful way to give yourself love in the form of a soothing touch. For some people, this gesture makes them feel uneasy. If you are one of them, I invite you to explore other ways of being there for yourself such as giving yourself a gentle squeeze or just focusing on your breathing. The next time you feel overwhelmed with emotion about fertility struggles (or anything difficult), try placing your hands over your heart, giving yourself a gentle hug, or just taking a few deep breaths. Say to yourself, "I love you and I don't want you to suffer." It is completely okay (and normal) to still have emotions through this coping process. I hope that you will experience less suffering and feel validated in treating yourself this way.

Self-Compassion and Fertility Struggles

Over the past decade, research on the effects of practicing self-compassion has grown at an exponential rate. Findings from numerous studies across many different populations—healthy adults, people struggling with chronic diseases, caregivers of terminally ill patients—have revealed that the more people practice self-compassion, the better their quality of life and well-being.

While one in eight women struggle with primary infertility (struggles to have a first child), up to 35 percent of women struggle with secondary infertility (struggles to have a child after having one or more).[4] In 2015, Raque-Bogdan and Hoffman[5] specifically explored the relationships among self-compassion, well-being, and infertility. This study is unique because the authors intentionally included women struggling with *both* primary and secondary infertility. Prior to this study, most research conducted was done so on women who were coping with primary infertility. Interestingly enough, researchers found similar levels of self-compassion, fertility-related stress, and subjective well-being among women struggling with primary or secondary infertility. Those who were struggling with primary infertility reported more social concern about their fertility struggles. While secondary infertility is still perceived as stressful, because these women have a child (or children) already, they feel less stigma as a result of their fertility struggles.

Drawing from my experiences, I felt so much pressure from society to get pregnant with my first child (real or imagined pressure . . . likely a combination!), I can definitely relate to these findings. I struggled so much when first pregnant to even say the words "I'm pregnant." Why? a) I couldn't believe it, and b) I was so scared about "jinxing" it. Once you have a child (or children), and in your heart you know that you are ready to have another baby, there is a different mindset—at least there was for me. When we were ready to start trying for a second baby, I was so scared about going back to that dark place—with the pressure of conceiving—that I refused to talk about it with anyone. I agreed to "see what would happen" before our scheduled frozen-embryo transfer, but I fully expected that we wouldn't be able to conceive naturally. Most times, whether you already have a child(ren) and desire to have more, you will be faced with questions such as "Oh, are you planning on having more kids?", "Would you like to have more? . . . Oh, I don't know if I'd want more," or "So, when is the next one coming? You can't have too much of a 'gap' between kids. Best to get it over and done with." What I have observed and learned through my personal experiences with this societal song-and-dance chatter is this: People mostly mean well. Sometimes they are simply curious to know if you will be having another baby, which, for many people, is genuine interest in and support of your family. However, in some cases, there is nothing genuine or heartfelt about those questions and statements. They are downright intrusive and demonstrate a lack of boundaries. Whichever category they fall into, tune into your heart and intuition and you'll know instinctively who truly cares and wants to hold space/be supportive versus who simply wants the scoop on the latest details in your life. I have learned a lot about what to say and not to say to people about family planning. I certainly don't always get it right, but I try to be as sensitive to a variety of life situations as possible.

How does self-compassion help with fertility struggles? For me, it was the core of getting through each day. Even as we began our journey with in-vitro fertilization (IVF), there were many ups and downs—mentally, physically, emotionally, and of course, spiritually—and I had to continually come back to my regular practice of self-compassion. What does the research say? Raque-Bogdan and Hoffman[5] further investigated the link between fertility struggles and well-being and found that self-compassion explained the connection between the *need for parenthood* (i.e., desire to be a parent) and subjective well-being. Self-compassion also explained the connection between *social concern* and subjective well-being. In other words, the more women struggling with fertility are self-compassionate, the better they are able to cope with their unfulfilled desire to become a mother, thus leading to better well-being. Additionally, practicing self-compassion also helps women cope with any social stigmas regarding their fertility challenges.

For me, being self-compassionate also helped defeat the comparison game, which is something we, as women, are notorious for and surprisingly good at. Ah, comparison, the thief of all joy, peace of mind, and of course, our self-esteem and worth—particularly as we are all on unique journeys to becoming mamas! It is interesting how often I find people comparing the length of their fertility journey with one another. Some friends feel awkward telling me they are pregnant after a shorter journey, and other people have been judgmental that my journey "only" spanned two years when they had been through longer as though there just "had to be" a decade-long struggle in our trying-to-conceive journey. I'm very mindful of the fact that for some, it can take years, decades in fact, before they conceive their firstborn, and then there are some who either conceive right away or in a few short months or years—all of which is completely *okay*. Each journey is unique to each individual/couple. No one thing is ever the same (except perhaps the feelings we each feel during our infertility struggles), so comparison and judgment are *not* the answer or antidote for this heartbreaking journey. Compassion is. I remember being extremely emotional after we had been trying for a few months. I share this truth because comparing how long your journey is to another person's is not helpful to anyone. Whatever you feel, you are justified in feeling that way. This is a key part of mindfulness: letting yourself feel what you feel. Over the past few years, I've connected with a number of women on the journey to conceive. Some are in tears after a few months of trying, while others are calm after having a miscarriage and then trying to conceive again a few months later. Everyone's feelings are totally normal and valid, and everyone's approach to managing their emotions will vary. I share this statement so that you don't judge yourself for feeling whatever you feel on your journey to conceive.

Many women struggling with infertility can be consumed by feelings of self-blame. It is very common for women to feel shame and significant

distress because they feel it is their fault for not being able to get pregnant. *If I could only lose X pounds, stress less, sleep more, eat healthier, do
the right exercises, meditate more, work less—then I would get pregnant.*
Interestingly, the research by Raque-Bogdan and Hoffman also showed
that self-compassion explains the connection between feelings of shame
and distress—such that practicing self-compassion helps one to cope with
feelings of shame so one experiences less distress. The authors suggest
that self-compassion likely protects women struggling with fertility from
feelings of self-blame.

What Worked for Me

During my journey, there were a few key strategies that I found helped
me cope with the ups and downs.

Self-care. Starting my day with one to twenty-five minutes of **me** time
was essential to being able to cope with the emotional roller coaster I was
on. Some days this was just one minute of checking in and bringing my
attention to my breathing; other days I would spend up to twenty-five
minutes just flowing through different yoga poses or stretches that my
body needed. Incorporating this aspect of mindful self-care helped me
shake off whatever had happened the day before and set me up for what
that day had in store. No matter where you are on your journey into
motherhood, I encourage you to carve out some time on a daily basis
to check in with yourself, see what you need (emotionally, physically,
mentally, spiritually, and socially), and create time in your day or your
week to fulfill that need. Practicing mindfulness and checking in with
yourself on a regular basis will help you take better care of yourself,
increase your ability to cope with stressful situations, and improve your
overall well-being.

Spiritual journey. I was incredibly lucky to be able to join a group of women on a year-long chakra journey course for the second year of my struggles with fertility. We met once a month for a full day to explore each of our chakras, practice yoga, and connect. This process gave me the opportunity to connect with an amazing group of women who were so supportive and helped me to really get to know myself—my body—what I truly needed. Through this course, I learned a style of meditation that enabled me to check in with my chakras and intentionally nourish or balance each one of them on a regular basis. This process empowered me by giving me such strong body awareness. Interesting enough, this is also when my dreams, which played a part in helping me find the answer to our fertility struggles, first began. While a chakra journey may not be the right fit for everyone, I encourage you to at least try to connect with some sort of group—be it religious, spiritual, or another type of support group, because recognizing that you are *not alone* can be powerfully comforting, particularly during the really tough times.

Social support. While I often did want to be alone when I was struggling with fertility, I also intentionally chose to spend time with people who really *got* me or at least tried to understand me or openly said they knew they couldn't truly empathize with what I was going through, but sat with me and provided unconditional love and support through my sadness. There were many people who did not fit into these three categories, and I had to limit my time with them. I often felt guilty for not wanting to see certain people, but when I practiced self-compassion, I knew that I needed to listen to my gut and take care of my needs while I was struggling. I encourage you to listen to your gut: Who makes you feel heard, validated, energized, or loved after spending time with them? Choose to spend more of your time with that person (or people) and know that true friends will always be there for you.

Self-Compassion and Motherhood

Self-compassion was a key part of helping me cope with my painful, lonely, and frustrating two-year journey with infertility. However, once I finally became pregnant, it was interesting to see how the resiliency and coping skills I developed while trying to get pregnant were still invaluable to me. We experienced numerous ups and downs early on in my pregnancy such as concerning test results regarding the viability of the pregnancy, and then once my son was born, further concerns and appointments with specialists—all of which turned out to be perfectly normal. However, as a new mama, it was such a stressful and emotional time to also be going through the added stress over the health of my baby. I was so grateful to have my strong faith in our journey, my belief that everything would work out, and my practice of checking in with myself and taking care of my needs so that I could take the best possible care of my sweet baby boy.

Fast forward to today. I am a grateful mama to two amazing boys and my fur baby. Driven by my journey, I now offer seminars and retreats to help women on the journey to conceive connect with each other, and I empower them as they continue on their journey. We have created these workshops to build on the power of the collective to help women feel seen and heard while providing them with space to talk about their journey. Each and every day, I work toward balancing the multiple needs of this wonderful life that I have chosen (and been blessed with). The roles of woman, wife, mother, daughter, friend, and researcher often have competing time demands that can be tricky to balance. My daily practice of self-compassion continues to help me to not only be the best version of myself in all of these roles but also to **enjoy the ride!**

If my story
helps one
woman, it will
give my journey a
purpose.

~Maria Blackley
@maria_carmel_

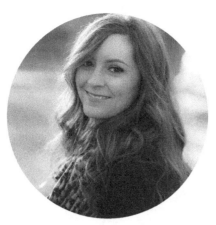

Maria Blackley

Warm-hearted, compassionate, resilient, fiercely determined, and genuine, Maria encompasses these traits while facing the challenges of infertility and pregnancy loss. As a strong-willed, active, and social child, she grew up knowing the importance of empathy, compassion, healthy habits, and standing up for what she believes in. She took these qualities and became a considerate woman with the desire for helping others while maintaining a healthy and active lifestyle. Maria feels life is just better if you feel better!

Maria met Dustin, the love of her life, at the young age of eighteen and together, they have grown into successful individuals creating a beautiful life with one another. They live in Vancouver, BC, and are both outdoor enthusiasts. You can often find them out camping, fishing, hiking, or walking with their adorable puppy! Maria is also a lover of wine, tea, chocolate, and a well-put-together charcuterie board! Maria and Dustin love spending time with their family and friends and are so grateful for the wonderful people in their lives.

Maria made the decision to be open and vulnerable with her own experience with infertility and pregnancy loss in hopes of inspiring and empowering other women and giving them the strength to get through a seemingly impossible time in their lives.

f   Maria Blackley
⊙   @maria_carmel_

~ To my husband, Dustin, who has kept me smiling even in the darkest times and has supported me every single day through this journey. I love you.

Sixteen

MY JOURNEY TO MOTHERHOOD—THE HARDEST THING LIFE HAS THROWN AT ME
Maria Blackley

"It is only in our darkest hours that we may discover the true strength of the brilliant light within ourselves that can never, ever, be dimmed."

~Doe Zantamata

Trying to become a mama is the hardest thing life has ever thrown at me. People are always telling me how strong I am when they hear my story; some days I feel strong and even brave, but other days I'm not even close. Staying positive in a battle only to be knocked down again and again has been hard but so crucial in navigating my way through our struggles. In addition, finding support through my village of family and friends is how I've gotten to where I am today, and I am forever grateful for each and every one of them. They say it takes a village to *raise* a child, but it can truly take a village to *create* a child as well. As a society, we rarely discuss topics such as infertility and pregnancy loss. In fact, it is one of the most taboo and stigmatized dialogues, but one that needs to be had nonetheless. No woman should be ashamed or feel like she is alone during this heartbreaking and exhausting journey. There was never a doubt that I would share my story with the world, it was just a matter of *how* and *when*. I wasn't able to talk about my struggle right away, but I knew when I was ready, I wanted to do so in a big way. My journey hasn't been harder or worse than anyone else's, just different. If my story helps even one woman find the strength to keep moving forward through her struggles, it will give my journey a purpose.

Growing up, I always knew I wanted to be a mama. When we set out to get pregnant, I had absolutely no idea how much this process would affect me—emotionally, mentally, physically, spiritually—mostly because I was so naïve and didn't realize how many barriers we would be up against. Like many women, I, too, was certain we would get pregnant quickly and without complications. I never thought for one second we would struggle. I have tried my best to stay positive through the ups and downs, but this journey has the ability to wear down a person. It breaks you down with each negative pregnancy test. You feel like less of a woman with every single hormone injection. Your heart is shattered in a million pieces with each pregnancy loss. You feel purposeless, guilty, ashamed, angry, embarrassed, and hurt. You feel alone and isolated as everyone around you starts the exciting journey of motherhood without you. You feel empty, heartbroken, and exhausted.

Our journey started two days before my twenty-ninth birthday. I found out I was pregnant after only two months of trying, so it came as a pretty big shock that it happened *that* quickly. It was a very confusing couple of days, but we were excited! It would be an amazing year. We were going to have our first baby! I didn't even skip my period. *How can you be pregnant and still get your period?* I didn't know it was possible. Everything was normal; however, afterward, I started to notice pregnancy symptoms.

The symptoms lasted for several days, and pregnancy crossed my mind, but I brushed it off, thinking it wasn't possible. When I finally decided to take a pregnancy test, much to my surprise, the test was positive. I did a second test, and it was positive as well. I waited a couple of hours and did a third test: positive, again. I was pregnant! Although a part of me still didn't believe it was true, I was excited to tell my husband. It's crazy how quickly you start thinking of baby names, wondering who your baby will look like, and planning out the nursery.

Just two days later, I woke up in the middle of the night with intense cramps. Throughout the night the cramps became worse, and I started bleeding. I knew something was very wrong, and on top of the confusion I already had, I knew bleeding wasn't a good sign. The excitement about being pregnant was short-lived and fear started to sink in. After several blood tests and two separate ultrasounds, the doctor was able to confirm that it was an ectopic pregnancy. He briefly explained what that meant and sent me to the emergency room immediately.

What is an ectopic pregnancy? In an ectopic pregnancy, the fertilized egg attaches (or implants) someplace other than the uterus, most often in the fallopian tube (which is why it is sometimes called a tubal pregnancy). In rare cases, the egg implants in an ovary, the cervix, or the belly. There is no way to save an ectopic pregnancy. It cannot turn into a normal pregnancy. If the egg keeps growing in the fallopian tube, it can damage or burst the tube and cause heavy bleeding that could be deadly.[1]

They performed more blood tests at the hospital while I waited in a small, claustrophobic room for what felt like days. Since I was a "good" candidate (I wasn't experiencing severe pain), they decided to treat my ectopic pregnancy with Methotrexate, a drug used in chemotherapy. Once injected, it would *slowly* dissolve the cells that made up the pregnancy, and my body would reabsorb them. *How morbid is that?*

I remember lying awake at night thinking about what was happening inside my body and being terrified that at any moment my tube would burst. It was traumatizing. After two weeks, the drug was finally working, so at that point I had to get a blood test done each week to watch my HCG (pregnancy hormone) until it was down to zero. It was the most depressing form of torture I'd ever gone through. Imagine watching something you want most in the world slowly and painfully getting farther away until any and all traces of it ever existing are completely gone.

The next several months were hard. I didn't feel like myself—physically, mentally, or emotionally. It felt like every other day we saw yet another pregnancy announcement on social media. Those were difficult. I felt very isolated. Learning that some of our best friends were pregnant was tough. Sometimes I would be overcome with feelings of guilt and jealousy, not because I wasn't happy for my friends or the women around me, but because I kept thinking, *why is this so easy for everyone else but us? Why me? Am I not motherly enough? Am I not worthy enough?*

A few months later we started trying to conceive again, but it still felt like an uphill battle, so I decided to try weekly acupuncture treatments as I heard they were really helpful. We spent hundreds of dollars on ovulation tests. I switched my diet completely—I eliminated gluten and processed foods, added healthy fats and oils, and totally stopped drinking alcohol. I started personal training twice a week. I ensured I was getting enough sleep and taking every vitamin and supplement that was recommended. We even took a relaxing trip to Hawaii, thinking that would help. After six months of acupuncture and everything else that went with it, we still had no luck, so we decided it was time to get a referral to a fertility clinic. It just didn't make sense. *We became pregnant so quickly the first time, so why was it taking longer now?* We didn't want to waste any more time in case there were other obstacles standing in the way of starting our family. Getting into the fertility clinic meant undergoing more tests, and every test result came back normal for the both of us. We still didn't have any answers.

After discussing our situation and test results with our reproductive endocrinologist (RE), we listened as she went over alternate options available to us at this point in our journey. After much consideration, we felt that in-vitro fertilization (IVF) was the next step for us, and we were fortunate enough to have that as an option. However, it still was an extremely tough decision to make. I was thirty years old, and although that is considered young, I put a lot of pressure on myself. *My clock was ticking. I wasn't getting any younger! I was ready to be a mama years ago. I didn't want to wait to start my family and then have it be too late!* I also felt in my gut that there was a reason why this wasn't happening naturally, and I felt like IVF was our best chance to start our family before it was too late. Through this process, I was so fortunate to make some new and very special friends, women who understood this journey because they had lived it or were living it. To be able to talk about my frustrations and share stories and feelings with someone else who had been there provided me with such a sense of comfort. It showed me that I was *not alone.* I was able to maintain a positive mindset because of the support system I had around me, the sisterhood I found within these women, and of course, the unconditional love and understanding shown to me by my spouse. It's extremely important to be comfortable with this decision and have a positive mindset going into IVF as it is far from easy.

In November 2017, we jumped into the IVF process. I did three hormone injections a day for ten days. My ovaries grew to the size of oranges but felt like bowling balls. I exercised internal strength on a level I didn't know I was capable of. I stayed optimistic throughout each day—some days I needed meditation to help me get there, but it was important to stay positive. My husband also handled this time in a way that made me love him even more. He did every injection for me and encouraged my strength in the times I felt weak. We were relieved to have had a successful IVF cycle that gave us two beautiful embryos—two chances at having the family we've dreamed of.

Near the end of February, I was feeling nervous but excited and *so* ready to get the next steps started. I was ready to get pregnant and become a mama! We waited for my cycle to start, and then we began the medications. After eighteen days, one embryo was transferred into my uterus. I was pregnant until proven otherwise! The next ten days were a test of patience like no other. I followed every health tip and trick, all the old wives' tales—I ate pineapple cores for five days, drank homemade broth and warm water every day, kept my feet warm, cut out caffeine, went for short walks, and listened to meditations to stay calm and relaxed. I pretty much did everything except lie with my legs up a wall. Eleven days after the embryo transfer, I went in for a pregnancy blood test and waited for a nurse to call with the results. It was one of the longest days of my life. I couldn't focus on anything; no book or TV show could distract me. Finally, at three o'clock in the afternoon, my phone rang. I was shaking. I heard those three words: "You are pregnant." I couldn't believe it. *FINALLY! IT WORKED! OMG! THIS IS IT!* I was so incredibly relieved because this meant our struggles were over and we were on our way to a new and exciting chapter in our lives.

We wanted to tell everyone! We told only our immediate family and closest friends because it was quite early in the pregnancy, and it's hard not to be overly cautious after our struggle to get there. We anxiously awaited the six-week ultrasound. I was feeling all the symptoms of pregnancy already, and at the six-week ultrasound we received the best news: The pregnancy was in the right spot, meaning it wasn't ectopic (which can still happen when doing IVF. Crazy!). We were also able to *see* the flickering of our baby's heartbeat. We felt pure joy! Our nurse told us that if they were able to see the heartbeat at the six-week ultrasound, the chances of miscarrying decreased drastically. We walked out of the doctor's office smiling ear to ear.

The next two weeks were long. We continued to stay cautiously optimistic. The medications were becoming a nuisance, and I was really looking forward to when I could stop the daily injections (at twelve weeks). We went in for another ultrasound at eight weeks to check the progress of development in our little baby. My gut felt uneasy as we drove to the doctor's office, just as I had felt for the six-week ultrasound. This time, however, I felt something was different, and the uneasiness never left me. We went to the room where the doctor set up the ultrasound. My husband held my hand as we anxiously waited to see the flickering on the screen again. It was then that we heard those soul-crushing words: "I can't find a heartbeat. I am so sorry. This pregnancy is not viable." My heart sank. My face heated up and my head spun. *This could not be happening.* This was the worst possible news we could have received. It didn't seem real. I thought it was a nightmare and wanted to wake from it. *I just did nine weeks of medications, we spent all this time and money, did all these tests . . . how is this happening? Again? Why us? This time wasn't supposed to end like this.* I started crying and couldn't stop. All the pain, all the grief, all the strength and courage—everything was too much to bear. The next few hours were a blur. I remember the doctor leaving the room. The nurse took us to another room and gave us pamphlets on miscarriages and very briefly went through our options. She advised me to stop taking all medications immediately. Still in shock, I cried uncontrollably. I was devastated. I was heartbroken.

It took a few days to process. After discussing all our options and realizing how equally horrible and risky they all were, we decided to wait and see if my body would miscarry naturally as that would be the least invasive and least risky option. I did end up miscarrying at home, about one week later. For those who understand, no explanation is needed. For those who do not understand, no explanation is possible.

We had a lot of questions as to why I miscarried since we knew the embryo was chromosomally normal, and we had been able to see the heartbeat at the six-week ultrasound. Again, I was left feeling like something else was going on in my body that we were not catching. My gut was telling me we were missing something. *This doesn't make sense. Everyone else can get pregnant and stay pregnant with minimal issues, so why is it so difficult for us?* Since we only had one embryo left, we were going to push to have more tests done. I wanted to know everything I could before our next embryo transfer, to set us up for the best possible success and to save ourselves from the heartache and devastation of another loss. Every day I focused on healing my mind, body, and soul and did my best to stay optimistic and hopeful. Although some days were harder than others, I knew deep down that I was meant to be a mama, and we *would* have the family we had always dreamed of. *We have fought way too hard and come so far; I will not give up now.*

Much to our surprise, we managed to get pregnant on our own, just a couple of months later. Unfortunately, the excitement was short-lived as it also ended in miscarriage. This loss made me feel numb. I felt shame for failing, again. I felt distrust in my body for not doing what it is supposed to be able to do so naturally. I felt anger toward the Universe for taking yet another baby away from us. *How are we here, in this place again? Why does my body hate me so much? This is not fair!*

We took a few months to heal and decide what the next steps would be for us. I went to a fertility retreat to connect with other women in similar situations. I wanted to try and regain some of my strength and hope as it had faded away, and I couldn't seem to find it again on my own. Losing three babies and having absolutely no idea why didn't give us much hope for any pregnancies working out in the future. The retreat was exactly what I needed to feel hopeful again. I learned how to be more compassionate with myself and that it's okay to get a second opinion. I regained some of my emotional strength and had the courage to keep moving forward. I knew I needed answers. I felt deep down that there had to be an explanation for these losses. A good friend's advice to me was to trust my gut, so I did. We decided to get a second opinion from a doctor in the United States whose practice focuses on Immunology Implantation Dysfunction (an autoimmune response to the embryo trying to implant into the uterus causing recurrent miscarriages).

The consultation went really well, and we had a lot of confidence in this doctor. For a couple of reasons, the doctor's advice was to do another cycle of IVF to "bank" more embryos as well as to do some additional testing to see if we could find out what was causing the miscarriages. We felt really good about this suggestion and decided to move forward. This protocol was different than the last time—it was much more intense—but it gave us hope that we would end up with more embryos so we could have a chance at the family we've always wanted. Everything went really well. My body responded to the medications and the doctors were able to retrieve several mature eggs. We also got back the test results confirming I did in fact have autoimmune issues that were causing my body to reject the pregnancies and miscarry. *FINALLY, SOME ANSWERS!* We now had a new protocol of medications for our next transfer. We had hope!

I was recovering well from the surgery and awaiting the doctor's call letting us know how many embryos we had from this cycle of IVF. Unfortunately, the call was not at all what we were expecting. We had no embryos. This cycle of IVF failed us. It left us with nothing but broken hearts! I was upset, angry, heartbroken, frustrated, and defeated. The reality of not being able to have biological children was becoming very real, and it absolutely crushed us.

Although our second cycle of IVF failed, we did not feel that it was a waste. We were able to get answers that explained why we had been struggling the last three years, and those answers came with a new medication protocol that would help our chances with our last and final embryo. Our chances were not high, but they were there. One thing I've learned through this entire experience, and often have to remind myself, is that it's NOT my fault. It's hard not to blame yourself, but the reality is, there is nothing I did or didn't do that caused infertility or miscarriages or failed IVF cycles.

As I sit here writing this chapter, I am beyond grateful to say that our last and final embryo transfer was successful, and I am currently twenty-six weeks pregnant! To say the medication protocol was intense would be an understatement. My life revolved around pills and injections every single day for the first twelve weeks during this pregnancy. No part of it was easy. It was a test of patience and my strength, once again, but worth every needle and bruise.

It's an absolute dream to finally have a successful pregnancy and feel those baby kicks and movements! At the same time, I am realizing just how difficult pregnancy after loss is. The fear and anxiety that we will lose this baby is real. Every ultrasound and every checkup has had me in a panic- and anxiety-ridden state. I am petrified of hearing those dreadful words from the doctor again. Every time I go to the bathroom, I am worried there will be blood. And going off all the medications felt the most terrifying. I was a bag of mixed emotions because although relieved, I was worried that's what was keeping our baby alive. From day one, we have broken down the pregnancy into small milestones and celebrate each one as it successfully passes. This practice has helped us focus on taking it one day at a time, which has made it less overwhelming. We waited a long time before telling friends and family because quite honestly, I struggled to even believe I was pregnant and that we were actually going to have a baby. I was hesitant to buy any maternity clothes or start our baby registry, and the thought of planning our baby shower was terrifying. I am not even sure when we will start the nursery. It's not that we aren't excited because we are over the moon, but after losing our first three babies, the fear has a way of sticking with you and not letting go. The further along we get in the pregnancy, the excitement definitely overshadows the fear, and I am learning that it's okay and totally natural to have a balance of hope and fear throughout a pregnancy after loss. Surrounding myself with my village, the most empathetic support system of family, friends, and various health care professionals who understand the array of emotions that go along with pregnancy after loss and know what it has taken for us to get here, has been everything. Finding your village is so important, to be heard, to validate your feelings, and to help maintain strength and a positive mindset when going through the roller coaster of infertility and pregnancy loss. I am forever grateful for everyone in our village who has supported us on this journey. We are doing our best to patiently await the arrival of our beautiful rainbow baby, the magical gift we will pull out of our storm.

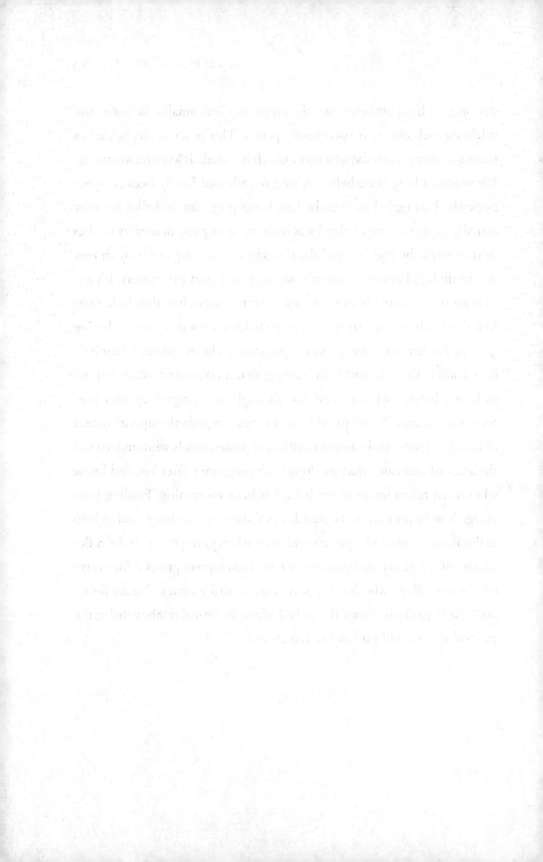

Through my eyes and heartbeat, my twins live on.

~ Shayroz Khosla
@Shayroz80

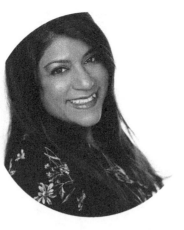

Shayroz Khosla

Shayroz graduated with a Bachelor of Science degree in nursing in 2003 and quickly discovered that nursing and serving others is her passion.

She has worked in the realm of organ transplant for the majority of her career. Her goal in life is to travel as much as possible and experience as many different cultures and religions as possible.

Becoming a wife and a mother changed Shayroz—it unleashed her inner confidence and helped her discover that she can do anything!

 Shayroz80

shayroz

@Shayroz80

~ To my children who inspire me to want more from this life.

Seventeen

MY JOURNEY IN THE RAW
Shayroz Khosla

*"And one day, she discovered that she was fierce,
and strong, and full of fire, and that not even
she could hold herself back because her passion
burned brighter than her fears."*
~Mark Anthony

It was one of those perfect moments—the smell of summer in the air, the sound of the canaries, and the feel of the grass as my daughter and I rolled around in it. I catch a glimpse of her smile and hear the sweet sound of her contagious laugh, and I think to myself, *How did I get here? How can this moment be one of the happiest moments of my life, and why am I bursting into tears?*

I think I was eighteen when the doctor told me I had polycystic ovarian syndrome (PCOS). He was so matter of fact when he told me I would most likely have trouble conceiving, and if I did, miscarriage would likely be the outcome. I didn't know how to react; I was shocked and stunned, feeling less and less like a woman with each word he said. He left the room while I felt like my world was ending. *How could I never be a mother? How will I face my family?* That doctor's visit shaped the course of my life—I never felt whole after that. I always felt (and still sometimes feel) like less of a woman.

Growing up, it was ingrained in me that a woman's fruitful womb was her greatest gift. In my culture, a woman is cherished and of great value because she *adds value* to her husband's family *by providing children.* A woman's beauty is based on her skin color: the more light skinned she is, the more beautiful. I was not born light skinned, and I tanned way too easily, and now my womb was not fruitful. My dreams of mother-hood just may have to remain a dream. I lost all value for myself. The reflection I saw in the mirror was nothing but a dark-skinned girl who could not have children. These thoughts ran rampant in my mind: *Who would ever want to marry me and love me? Will my family accept me when I tell them I have PCOS?*

My dating life was like a CD on repeat. In comes said guy. I like him, I tell him I may never be able to have kids, and then out the door he goes. I met a guy online, someone who I initially thought I could settle down with, and whaddaya know? He was cheating on me! After that relation-ship ended, I took a long break from dating to rediscover myself, find meaning in my life as a single professional, and tune into my happiness.

Fast forward a few years. I finally met my husband—I fell in love with him the moment I locked eyes with him. I remember thinking to myself, *How am I going to pick myself up when I tell him I may never be a mother and he leaves me?* I waited for the longest time to tell him my secret. I wanted to cherish every moment I had with him—his touch, his embrace, his smile, the way he smelled—until one day I finally shared my truth with him. Sam looked right at me and said, "I want to be with *you.* Then it's just the two of us and no kids." It was at that moment I truly knew what love felt like. He wanted *me*; he didn't care that I was dark or that I may not conceive. He loved me for me. I had never felt that before—complete acceptance. It wasn't long after we were married that I insisted we try for children.

Several rounds of Clomid, two failed intrauterine inseminations, and finally in-vitro fertilization (IVF): I didn't know how intense and all-consuming these treatments could be. The highs and lows were so intense. The mood swings, hot flashes, breakouts, and growth of body hair in places I'd rather not mention all combined with the worst news you could get from medical professionals: "Your pregnancy test is negative." My relationship with my friends and family changed, and any close friendships I had built at work completely broke down. I started to *survive* in a job I once loved, which only added to the stress of everything else. I became a fragment of who I once was. My whole life was about my treatments and medications. I stopped everything I did for *myself*. I stopped doing yoga, I stopped reading (the only material I ever read now revolved around how to make my fertility treatments a success), I avoided any social commitments, and I stopped taking care of myself. I felt so alone.

Finally, after multiple rounds and treatments and a whole roller coaster of emotional turmoil later, we were pregnant. I was admitted to emergency when we first found out the pregnancy test was positive. Complications from the IVF treatments resulted in me having ovarian hyperstimulation syndrome (OHS). I gained twenty-five pounds in ascites, and my lungs filled with fluid. I was vomiting every few minutes, and the pain of the fluid was so intense. It hurt to breathe and walk, but it didn't matter. *I was pregnant.* We were so happy, and I started feeling more like myself again. Our fertility doctor told us we were pregnant with twins—a boy and a girl. We decided to name our babies Safeel and Saraa. Safeel means "happiness" and Saraa means "pure." Pure happiness indeed. Words could not explain how happy I felt and how much love I felt for my babies.

We bought a house, and as we were getting ready to move (I remember it was a Sunday because Sam was leaving to play hockey), I told him that something didn't feel right. Reluctantly, I tried to calm myself and took a nap. I had an ultrasound scheduled the next day and told myself that everything was fine; I was just being crazy. The next day Sam surprised me at work by picking me up to go to my appointment together. The ultrasound technician let us hear the babies' heartbeats, and we looked at each other and smiled; everything was worth it if it meant we got to have them. Suddenly, however, the technician stopped talking to us and abruptly left the room. The radiologist came into the room and the look on his face told me more than his words. He told us to go to labor and delivery right way—my cervix had shortened, and I could go into labor at any time. When we arrived at the hospital, many doctors went in and out of the room, each one telling me different things. I was so confused. Finally, my ob-gyn came to see me and told me there was no hope left. She said we could try bed rest with the hope to carry this pregnancy for a few more weeks to give my babies a chance at survival. I went for another ultrasound the next day and the doctor told me that Twin A's (my son's) legs were out of my cervix and labor was inevitable. I burst into tears. She gave me a gentle reminder that I could not cry as it would bring on my labor and there was still a chance that Twin B may stay in my uterus and my cervix would close after Twin A was delivered.

I stayed on bed rest for several days. I didn't cry; instead, I prayed every minute I was there. The bleeding started, and so did the contractions. They moved me to the delivery room, and with my husband and family by my side, the contractions grew stronger and stronger. The pain was too much to bear at times. When it was time to push, I told everyone to leave except Sam. I didn't want to push, but the nurses kept forcing me. I don't know what hurt more—the labor or knowing at least one of my babies would die. I would deliver my son but felt that my daughter may have more time in my womb.

With each push and each contraction went another piece of my soul. Then it happened—*his* body came out of mine, silent. No crying, no wriggling, nothing. Just pure silence. No one said anything. The doctor told me Saraa's sac had fallen too, and I would have to push again soon. The tears burned like acid down my face, and within minutes, I was pushing again. Her lifeless body came out of mine as well. They were too small to live; I couldn't save them. My body had failed. I failed.

It was the first time I saw my husband break down the way he did. I had forced him to do fertility treatments and brought this pain onto him, and now I couldn't help him. My world fell silent. I was there, but only physically. Emotionally and mentally, I could no longer hear anything anymore. The doctors and nurses rushed around me and my parents and sister came to the hospital in the morning, but they were all blurs to me. What I remember the most clearly, however, was my father telling me that my twins were defective and wanting me to reassure him I could have more children. It was so tough because I had no idea if I could. I wanted to scream, "Get out!" Instead, I swallowed my screams and my tears. I couldn't look anyone in the eye, and I certainly didn't want anyone to touch my babies' bodies. They were too delicate and small.

The grief nurse came in to talk, but I just wanted her to leave as I laid on the delivery bed with my babies' bodies next to mine. I didn't need her. At least, I didn't know how much I needed her. I wish even now that I was more open with her. The hospital sent a photographer to take pictures of my beautiful babies; I wished I had agreed to be in the pictures. It's a regret I still have. I hope they don't ask the next bereaved mom whether she wants to be in the picture. The photographer should click her picture with her stillborn child.

I held my still babies and smelled them. I tried to memorize every inch of them. Their little bodies were so limp and lifeless, yet so beautiful. I gave so many kisses to my babies who never lived, yet lived. I held their bodies for the last time. I kissed them and hugged them. I whispered all my hopes and dreams for them in their ears. I told them how loved and wanted they were and how I hoped they felt this, wherever their souls may be. I held my husband's hand, along with two teddy bears the nurses gave us, and left behind the sounds of all the babies crying and the screams of laboring women.

The next day we visited the babies at the funeral home. I held them both in my arms; they were ice cold, and no matter how tightly I held them, they never warmed. Their eyes never opened, their little hands never to hold mine. I never heard their cries or giggles. It really sank in that they were dead. I cried harder than I ever had in my life. *They died, they died, they died* and there was literally nothing I could do. I just wanted to break everything, scream, and cry. As I walked out of the funeral home with my body that still looked pregnant, I understood what real sorrow felt like.

The funeral was the next day. That morning of the funeral, it started snowing out of the blue, and it was so cold. My mosque leaders lowered the little coffin, and as it met the ground, the sun started to shine. I believed in that moment my babies' souls had found peace. Our friends came from all around to be with us for the funeral. It meant so much to me. Later in the evening, they all came over to spend time with us, but I just couldn't be there. I tried to stay for as long as I could, and then my mother-in-law started talking about when she had had my husband and her birth experience. This led to my family and friends sharing their birth experiences. I could feel the choke hold tightening around my neck and chest. I just couldn't be there, so I left. That was my breaking point. I cried and cried and then eventually fell asleep. I had no idea when everyone left. My bed became my island, my safe place.

I pushed Sam away. I wanted him to leave me and marry someone else. I don't know what would have happened to me if he left, but he didn't. He gave me so much love and understanding, which made me feel even worse. I would look in the mirror and hate what I saw: my postpartum body, breasts that leaked milk for months, and depression. Six weeks later, I had to go back to work. I had to face all the pregnant ladies, hear about how my two other colleagues had healthy babies while I was off, all the while grieving the loss of my two angels. I remember how numb I felt having to explain that I wasn't pregnant anymore. It was a very exhausting time in my life.

I was determined to conceive again as soon as possible. I truly thought conceiving would take all my pain away. But through treatment after treatment, my body kept failing me. We finally decided to do a fresh round of IVF, and Sam was firm that it would be our last try. Finally, I was pregnant again. I was happy, anxious, and terrified. I was so afraid that my pregnancy would end. I tried to be detached from this pregnancy, but that didn't last long. As soon as I heard the baby's heartbeat, I was so in love. We were also relieved that Sophia was a single pregnancy.

It took a team of medical professionals and five long months of bed rest to keep me pregnant. Finally, my beautiful daughter, Sophia Savitri Khosla, was born. I didn't hear her cry when she was born, and I panicked until I finally heard that first cry. I held her, took in her scent, and was so in love. At that moment, I thought back to my twins; Sophia's body was so warm and pink, and so alive, while the twins had not been. Our nurse, a good friend, and our doctors were happy and joyful with Sophia; with my twins, it had been so quiet and dreary. Such different experiences.

The next few weeks were a spiral of emotions. I had been so sad and anxious for so long, and now, all of a sudden, I was supposed to be happy, but I didn't know how to be. As luck would have it, I couldn't breastfeed. After my first pregnancy, my milk had come in with a vengeance and was relentless. Now I felt like my body was failing again. But I've learned that fed is fed, and fed is best, and my toddler is healthy and smart.

I have finally come to a point where I believe I have value, and I have a lot to offer—a lot of love, a lot of kindness, and a lot more of myself. It doesn't matter what the color of my skin is or what kinds of fertility challenges I face. I still dream of my twins' butterfly kicks in my womb, the sound of their heartbeats, their smell, and how they both looked so much like their father. I wake up and realize they aren't with me. Reality sinks in along with her good friend panic, and I can't catch my breath. I wake up and know that I need to be the best mother to my daughter and wife to my husband, and that I live for three. Through my eyes and my heartbeat, my twins live on. They experience everything I experience: the sweet kisses my daughter gives me, the tight hugs, and all the fun we have.

There are days that are still so tough—all the firsts that I have missed and will continue to miss. This year, my twins would have started kindergarten. I cried, took a day off work and wallowed in self-pity, and laid flowers on their little grave. I wonder how life can be so beautiful and yet so ugly? How can having children be so easy for so many and so hard for me? I lost so much of myself on my journey to motherhood: my career ambitions and so many people who I once cherished. But I gained so much too. I get to experience the best adventure: raising my daughter. Through being a mother, I found myself again. I never knew I could love someone as much as I love my babies. My children have impacted my life so much and changed me for the better.

I truly have no advice to give to anyone going through fertility treatments except this: *Do whatever you feel is right for you, Mama.* I wish someone would have kept reminding me that *I am important*, and I need to take care of me. I need to be kind and patient with myself and remind myself every morning how amazing and beautiful my body is. I tell my daughter every morning how beautiful her body is and if she wants, she can change the world. She is smart, compassionate, and beautiful. I hope she grows up and knows this is her life and her journey, and whatever she decides, I will be right by her side to support her unconditionally.

Whatever your journey is, no matter how you feel some days, please know you've got this, Mama. You are enough. Don't ever underestimate how strong you are and how much courage you have!

Intuition: the place between head and heart, nurtured and informed by both: where magic dwells.

-Leisha Laird
@flourishwellnesscentre

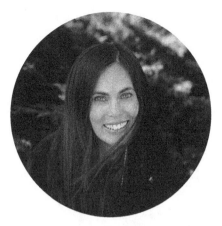

Leisha Laird

Leisha Laird is a Doctor of Traditional Chinese Medicine (TCMD), a registered acupuncturist, and owner of Flourish Wellness in Calgary, Alberta. She supports couples (in collaboration with natural, IVF, and fertility treatments) as they navigate through fertility, pregnancy, and childhood. Her practice focuses on a healthy mind, spirit, and body, empowering individuals and families to Be Well. Leisha is a regional chair and an active board member of the Obstetrical Acupuncture Association (OBAA), and she works closely with the midwifery and doula communities in both Alberta and British Columbia as well as in developing countries.

Leisha's practice centers on nurturing her patients' wellness through intuition, grounded research, nutrition, and acupuncture. She works collaboratively and compassionately with clients, offering space to be seen and heard while inviting them to flourish in all areas of their life. She meets her clients with empathy, allowing their personal experience to be met with an expanded sense of self, knowing, calm, and confidence to move forward.

Leisha feels most deeply fulfilled when in connection with nature, animals, and those she holds dear. She values clarity, integrity, and the courage to be vulnerable. Leisha is grateful to be on this journey with her big-hearted, humor-filled husband, and their two sparkly children who keep it all mighty real.

 flourishwellness.ca

@flourishwellnesscentre

~I dedicate this chapter to the incredible women I have had the privilege to walk beside in my practice. Their courage to be vulnerable, their trust and their openness to expand. And to all the magical children who have arrived earthside into these families.

Eighteen

WHERE MAGIC DWELLS
Leisha Laird

*"I've learned that people will forget what you
said, people will forget what you did, but people
will never forget how you made them feel."*
–Maya Angelou

I remember traveling in Bhutan a few years into our journey of hoping to conceive our daughter. Prayer flags were everywhere. The monk traveling with us shared that each time they blew in the wind, the blessings bestowed on them are activated, their inherent intention sparked. Some flags were hung for prosperity, some for luck or karma, others to help loved ones pass on. Traveling through this spiritual country and grounding landscape felt magical. It created a sense of spaciousness, allowing me to be present. To listen.

Something about a particular set of prayer flags we passed made me pause and take a picture. That evening, when we arrived back at the hotel, I had a message from my parents, telling me my aunt had passed away. Months later, back home in Canada, I was sitting with my cousin who shared the actual time of my aunt's passing. I'd brought with me a print of the flags I'd photographed to give her. On it was a time stamp.

I'd snapped the picture two minutes before she passed.

Listening to that inner whisper in Bhutan seemed to come more easily; the reminder of still not being pregnant somehow quieted by the distraction of travel. I could be present, make things happen, bounce back from adversity and hear my intuition loud and clear when life was mostly headed in a direction I desired. The challenge came in those moments where my timing and the Universe's timing looked different. The push-pull this created made *getting pregnant* the end goal. Yet this is not how life's biggest lessons work. Action and handwork, which served me well through my life, were exactly what needed to be balanced with something else in this world of the unknown. I couldn't power through this one. I had to find a way to grow and expand, even as I embraced this foreign place of surrender.

My journey was centered around this idea. Trusting both the seen and unseen; known and unknown. Trusting myself, and in a master plan bigger than myself.

Having challenges conceiving is a year-round consumption. There are holidays for a few days when you have moved through the disappointment of getting your cycle to when you start focusing on the next chance to conceive. There are questions to fill your time with: *Do I need to eat differently? When should we be intimate? Will that work with our schedules? More meditation?* More and more to-dos and not much room for flow or joy. Certainly not the advertised notion that pregnancy happened easily.

Inevitably, someone would offer, "Just relax," or announce, "I got pregnant just walking past my husband," or worse, "Maybe it isn't meant to be." Or one of the juicier ones, "I had a friend going through IVF; her embryos were tested and most of them came back with a high propensity for genetic issues. It really changes when you hit thirty-five." I caught myself thinking, *this wasn't fair. Why me?* But life isn't fair, so why *not* me? We all have our challenges, and this was one of mine, as much as it turned out to be an opportunity.

Initially, I wanted to yell, distance myself from those who didn't have the capacity to hold empathy and awareness, who made it about themselves whether they meant to or not. It brought up a deep vulnerability that felt too raw to be volleyed around by just anybody. Somewhere deep in my core, fertility equated to being a strong female; a mother; my purpose. Intellectually, I knew that notion bore no truth. Some of the most powerful women and mentors in my life had no children. *So what was this shame and resentment I felt? Why was I so triggered by the comments of others?*

Fertility has no bearing on the path to enlightenment. We all face joy and challenges, they just show up in different ways. My challenge was to separate fertility from my sense of worth; the belief I wasn't enough. To realize I was a powerful, nurturing woman—children or not.

Author Brené Brown once said in an interview: "People aren't sucking on purpose to piss me off. They are doing the best they can. So what boundaries need to be in place (by me) for me to stay in my integrity and make the most generous assumptions about you?"[1] In other words, this generosity can't exist without my healthy boundaries. Bells went off in my head. There was another option to resentment? *This* was my chance to make generous assumptions about those few people in my life by whom I felt most critically judged. Talk about fertile soil to grow this awareness and create healthier boundaries. A chance to meet them with compassion and empathy, not resentment. To stop my eye roll before it began.

I realized I looked at boundaries as a defense against what felt threatening instead of as support. It was an exhausting and disempowering perspective. Choosing agency over resentment meant it was okay to say *no* to a baby shower and make a different choice. I wasn't being selfish, quite the opposite—I was supporting myself in order to hold my own integrity. Putting *Self* in the first position and casting away any shame that might otherwise surround my decisions. Thus, I could both feel excited for a pregnant friend *and* disappointment that I was not.

Boundaries began to feel more like radar. When I began to feel defensive, my muscles tightening, holding my breath, I took a moment to reflect on *what* was bothersome about the situation. In those moments, I offered, "Let me get back to you on that." This response served to instantly downgrade the storm threatening to sweep me, and instead allowed space and time to check in with what felt right rather than what I thought I *should* do, say, or think. In that moment, I offered myself the same grace I offer the women who move through my clinic: *I see you. I feel you. You are enough. You are powerful. You've got this.*

Three years into our journey to get pregnant, we were traveling through Burma. At the time I was reading a book called *Left to Tell* by Immaculee Ilibagiza. It's the true story about her journey through the Rwandan genocide and, more remarkably, her ability to forgive those who had taken part in its atrocities. I was struck by her absolute faith in something bigger, even amidst the dire situation she found herself in. The morning after finishing her book, I went on a hike deep into the countryside with my husband. It was early in the morning, and the last village we had walked past was fifteen minutes behind us. Surrounded by trees and rolling hills, I was reflecting on Immaculee's message when I noticed a little boy walking toward me. It was one of those moments when you feel someone looking deeply within you. *Through you.* He smiled, then silently, gracefully, handed me a flower, his eyes dancing excitedly. Then he walked away. I knew at that moment we would have a child. It wasn't a fleeting feeling, but a deep knowing, one I heard loud and clear.

Trust, Leisha, this will happen. Have faith and stay open. Don't forget the magic around you. Though they remembered the flower, neither my husband nor our guide remembers seeing the boy.

Two months later we were pregnant with our daughter, whom we named Grace.

Time is a funny thing, though. When you have a child and look at events in the rearview mirror, it feels like it happened so fast, even though the process took years. Now fully in the mix of parenting, on the other side of the ups and downs of hopeful conception, it's easier to reflect on the lessons of letting go, of trusting, the deep well of emotions that come with having no control, you begin to think, *Okay, check—I've got that lesson. Next?*

Then the next opportunity to conceive happens—or, more accurately—doesn't. All of a sudden I'm right back in that swamp of emotions: the stuck-ness, the panic, the feeling of being in reverse. The ease of going with the flow of the Universe is suddenly challenged, and time comes into play once more . . . whether it's timing my cycle, ovulation, or time in relation to everyone around me moving in a direction I so want to share but feel powerless to control.

One of my greatest teachers, Sher, came into my life as we were five years into the effort to welcome a sibling into our family. She challenged me on many things, one of which was the words I was using in my vocabulary. What energy they carried. How to create more integrity between my words, intentions, and actions. In fact, she was so serious about it, she said that every time I used one of her *no-go words* in writing or speech, I was to drop down and do ten burpees—no matter where I was. It was occasionally funny, though often incredibly awkward.

Try. This was the word that tripped me up more than any other word she gave me. When it comes to conception, "try" is the most common word used. *We are **trying** for a child. I am **trying** IVF.* Sitting with that word, I began to feel its weakness, the desperation and victim energy it elicited in me. It felt the opposite of empowering and trusting.

These words rarely challenge me when life is flowing, in those magical moments when my faith is immovable. Rather, they show up when I am stuck. Not trusting. In a tug of war with the Universe because I think I absolutely know better. These words are my checkpoint; when I hear them, I know what I need to do: expand what makes me feel connected. For me, that is solitude, walks in nature, time with my heart family and spending time in my body—mediation in whatever form speaks to me at that moment.

Unsurprisingly, all these moments share a common theme: joy, connection, and vulnerability.

At this point, I had been supporting and guiding women on their fertility journeys for eight years as a doctor of Chinese medicine. Professionally, I encourage my clients to look at both Western and alternative medicines, blending and mixing to the betterment of both, rather than strictly adhering to one discipline or another. The fact is that there is no one or right way to conceive. Whether becoming pregnant spontaneously, via IVF, waiting it out, alternative measures, surrogacy, egg donor, sperm donor, adoption, same-sex couple—there are so many ways to grow a family.

One afternoon I was at the fertility clinic, working with a couple going through an embryo transfer after an IVF cycle. My client was a researcher and spent her time in labs so was familiar and comfortable with the world of science. The embryologist came over and shared that the couple's embryo quality was poor, he didn't expect much from the transfer, and he didn't think any other embryos would make it to freezing. After he left, the woman asked me what I thought. I shared that some of the *worst*-looking embryos had created the most beautiful babies in my clinic.

This is the point where science stops and something else takes over. Eight days later she had a call from the embryology lab to say that, to their surprise, three embryos had gone to the blast stage and were frozen. She ended up pregnant and had a beautiful healthy girl from that cycle.

The second incredible gift of that situation was my recognition that I had created this condition within myself that if I were going to go with the flow of the Universe, I needed to not force conception, which in my mind meant no to IVF. I was placing a hard stop on IVF, equating it with failure. Not controlling didn't mean not taking action. Removing this condition was liberating.

At the time, I'd often have clients ask me how I could be fully present, empathetic, and supportive of them moving through fertility challenges since I was going through my own. The fact is, I *was* them, in so many ways—how could I not be empathetic? Indeed, walking alongside as they became pregnant, sharing this honest and vulnerable space with another, felt expansive and deeply connecting. The joy, hope, and expansion these experiences offered and continue to offer—this service to another—is as great a gift I could ever receive and a powerful counter to doubt and fear. I grew as much as they did.

No one goes through the highs of finding out they are pregnant to the lows of moving through miscarriage or loss by choice. Yet I realized, both watching women and experiencing it myself, that something grew from this dark place.

Grit.

The ability to get back up and move forward after another miscarriage, a failed IVF cycle, another month of not conceiving—it built resilience. I wasn't the one controlling the outcome of this journey to expand our family, yet not controlling didn't mean not taking action. I wasn't just along for the ride. As Rick Hanson, PhD suggests, "True resilience fosters well-being, and an underlying sense of happiness, love, and peace."[2] Remarkably, as you internalize experiences of well-being, that builds inner strength, which in turn, makes you more resilient. Well-being and resilience promote each other in an upward spiral. Grit and resilience are what this journey offered in spades.

Six years into our journey to have a second child, we were out visiting my in-laws on the Southern Gulf Islands in British Columbia. This is rain-forest country, and there was a particular grove we walked through regularly. My husband, daughter, mother-in-law, and I were headed back through the forest to the house when we came upon a soaring cedar, and at its base, a small wooden door. A fairy door. When the door opened, messages in a jar, crystals, and fairy objects glimmered inside. Our daughter took out a message and read it aloud: "Just because you can't see it," she said with the earnestness only a six year old can exude, "doesn't mean it isn't there or isn't real."

Most days forests feel magical to me; however, that day it felt like there was something else in the air. As we continued our walk, I found myself reflecting on trust, playing with the idea that it was like the path we were walking on. Though I couldn't see what lay ahead, *what* might happen if I simply trusted in the possibility that whatever *is* around the corner could be even better than what I'd wish it to be? That I might float along the middle of the river of my life instead of bouncing from bank to bank. Struggling between my head and its endless thoughts, my heart and its intention. And the place between head and heart nurtured and informed by both. *That's* where intuition lives and where I find the magic.

Further along the path, we met a ninety-three-year-old Scottish woman. She said she lived on the island and had been there for many years. She had a twinkle and wisdom in her eyes, which invited our daughter to ask if she knew the fairy house. "Why yes! Do you believe in fairies?" Our daughter and I responded "Absolutely!" She paused, then said, "I want to tell you something, and I don't ever want you to forget it. Fairies exist. Just because you can't see something doesn't mean it isn't there. Your job is to not forget that. Don't let adults tell you otherwise and keep that belief as you age. I am ninety-three, and there is magic all around us. Don't stop believing and seeing." We all stood in awe as she captured our attention and hearts.

My mother-in-law walks that small path regularly; she's never seen that magical lady, before or since.

I have a deep respect for Western medicine and all it can offer, especially in the fertility realm. Yet with all of the focus on hormone levels, age, embryo quality, the constant questions and thoughts of "Where in my cycle am I?" and "Is this going to happen?"—questions leading to more questions, muddying the water of intuition, that pool of knowing, best kept in stillness, only fully realized in peaceful apprehension. Some things simply can't be explained by science, blood tests, or embryo quality. These moments, what I call *magical moments*, grounded me in my body, opening a deep sense of trust in myself along with a vibrant peace—come what may.

We welcomed our son into the world nine months later.

I choose who I share these experiences with. They are profound. Not everyone can hold them with me. I share them here because they're what brought me from mind energy to heart energy, then back again, to a place of balance, roughly in the middle—where intuition resides. Where knowing lives. Where magic dwells.

Despite its endless stream of thoughts, my mind wasn't my enemy. Its guidance through the years has delivered me to many wise choices, in all aspects of my life.

The Universe operates according to its own timeline and ethereal principles, which can be at turns as remarkable as they are maddening. Looking back, both of our children came with their own perfect timing, for us, for them, and for our family as a whole. And our son's birth? The parking stamp showed we were at the hospital for 5 hours and 55 minutes, exactly.

Final Thoughts

FEATURING

Sabrina Greer

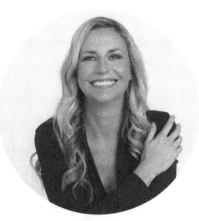

Sabrina Greer

Sabrina is a 2x bestselling author and the mastermind behind this popular motherhood guidebook series, which has been coined *"Chicken Soup for the Mama Soul"* by numerous publications. She is the founder of YGTMAMA Inc., a company built on love and focused on inclusive resources and opportunities for mothers. Sabrina also curates a popular collective blog space and is the host of *You've Got This, Mama—The Podcast.*

Sabrina is an aspiring philanthropist who knew from a young age that there was no box for her to comfortably fit into and that her life needed to be one by design. After ten years of traveling, modeling, and volunteering overseas, she found home base back in Ontario, Canada, where she was born and decided to earn her degree in education and developmental psychology to accredit her world-changing efforts. It did not take long for her to realize that her superpowers lay in entrepreneurship and coaching others to discover their potential. She is a certified NLP practitioner and clarity coach for mamas. She is the Eastern Canada Ambassador for *Mamas for Mamas*, an award-winning charity that supports mothers in crisis and provides ongoing support to low-income mamas and their kids. Their mission is a future in which no mama or child is left behind.

When she is not writing or attempting to save the world, you will likely find her exploring her wild feminine in nature, near water or momming hard to her three awesome boys: Oliver (13), Sterling (4), and Walker (2).

 ygtmama.com

You've Got This, Mama (ygtmama)

@ygtmama

~ To every single imperfect mama out there, I see you and love you. To my village, thank you for showing up and loving me in all my imperfections. To my Hubs, thank you for putting up with my wild visions and helping me stretch through the growing pains of both business and life. To my boys, thank you for being my mirror and showing me both the good and the ugly; I am so grateful for your lessons and unconditional love. To my parents, for giving me life in more ways than just the physical.

Health. How do you view and define health now, after reading the chapters in this book? What I have discovered on my journey through the stories shared here is that health, while subjective and differently interpreted, is actually the most important thing we have. Really, it's all we've got. Without optimal health, soundness of body, mind, and spirit, we cannot properly care for ourselves or our families. I write this now, curled up in bed, *sick as a dog* as they say, and I've had to ask for help. Dun, dun, dun . . . the core of where all mom guilt derives—having to ask for help: help to prepare meals, help to watch our young children, help with basic, seemingly effortless tasks. *I'm supposed to be superhuman, aren't I? I don't have time for this. I have taken all the proper steps in avoiding this, how could this happen? How could I be so weak?*

I rarely get sick anymore. I eat well, exercise regularly, take naturopathic supplements. I get adequate rest, drink lots of water, live in a clean environment. I have most of my emotional and mental faculties in check and have a spiritual practice that I enjoy daily. However, I'm not immune to everything. I am human. We are all human, Mama. The kids bring things home from school and daycare. Croup, pink eye, lice, colds, flus—it's inevitable. What's important when you do get taken out of commission is to be kind and gentle with yourself. Put that to-do list away and **ask for help**. Know it is okay to ask for help, to *need* someone else for a change.

I'm very fortunate and grateful to live in a country where medicine is a human right and mostly free. Where alternative medicine is used openly alongside Western medicine to create optimal health for their citizens. Is it flawless? No, but it's a start. Spending nearly ten years living abroad and volunteering in impoverished, third-world countries opened my eyes to the level of gratitude I need to express toward this fact. We so often take the simplest of things for granted. We have clean water to drink, ease and accessibility to a variety of foods, and a plethora of information, education, and other resources at our fingertips. I am also highly empathetic to our friends directly south of the border (many of the authors in this book). The medical bankruptcy statistics in the United States are staggering. It costs thousands of dollars just to deliver a baby in the US, and that is without any interventions or complications.

So is unhealthy synonymous with being sick? Disease, if you break down the word, equals dis-ease. To be ill is to be in a constant state of dis-ease. It is a vicious cycle when you think about it. What causes dis-ease? Stress. Anxiety. Busyness. And of course, repressing all your emotions. Feeling like you *have* to do it all alone. Feeling like you cannot ask for help for fear of what *they* think. *Who are they, anyway?* These factors can make you physically ill, and being physically ill can make you stressed and anxious. Add motherhood into the mix and it becomes next level. I've said it before, but motherhood is the only job where you can't call up your boss and take a sick day or a mental health day. Young children do not yet have the capacity or understanding to be compassionate or empathetic to the needs of others. To be a mother is to constantly live in a state of selflessness, not just toward your children and family, but toward yourself as well. Yes, we have a responsibility to our children to keep them safe and healthy, but we also have a responsibility to ourselves: to keep ourselves well—body, mind and spirit. We have heard the saying that *you cannot pour from an empty cup* and the analogy of the oxygen mask: Make sure you put your mask on before helping others; you are no good to anyone if you are dead. A dear friend and original co-author, Sunit Suchdev, once told me, "Self-care should not be a *thing* that we do or need to make time for, self-care should be non-negotiable, something that just is." This comment made me rethink a lot of things. Self-care is the root of optimal health; it needs to be woven into the tapestry that is motherhood. It is essential. Taking care of yourself, whatever that means for you, however that looks to you, is an absolute must.

Throughout this book we hear from a lot of mamas with different stories, opinions, backgrounds, and professional experiences, but the common thread throughout is this: We are somehow all cut from the same cloth, and we are in this together. To be healthy means to be the best version of yourself, your WHOLE self. Achieving this soundness will surely look different for everyone, but hopefully, this book will give you some ideas on where to start. I think the most important thing to remember, always, is that you are never alone, and wherever you are in your health story, **you've got this, Mama**.

End Notes

Introduction by Sabrina Greer

Page 3

> 1. Press Releases. (n.d.). Retrieved from https://globalwellnessinstitute.org/press-room/press-releases.

Page 5

> 2. Clegg, B. (2013, January 27). 20 amazing facts about the human body. Retrieved from http://www.theguardian.com/science/2013/jan/27/20-human-body-facts-science.

Chapter 1 by Daphne Kostova

Page 21

> Opening quote:
> Louise L. Hay Quotes. BrainyQuote.com, BrainyMedia Inc, 2019. https://www.brainyquote.com/quotes/louise_l_hay_178049, retrieved October 16, 2019.

Chapter 2 by Jennifer Kaley Smits

Page 35

> Opening quote:
> https://www.goodreads.com/author/quotes/73478.Jill_Churchill, retrieved October 16, 2019.

Chapter 3 by Stephanie Moody

Page 47

Opening quote:
Serrallach, Oscar. (2018). The Postnatal Depletion Cure.
London, Great Britain: Sphere

Page 48

1. Lee, Diane. (2017) Diastasis Rectus
Abdominis - A Clinical Guide For Those Who Are Split Down the
Middle. Surrey, BC: Learn, Pg. 10.
2. Johnson, Kimberly Ann. (2017). The Fourth Trimester: A
postpartum guide to healing your body, balancing your emotions &
restoring your vitality. Boulder, CO: Shambala, Pg. 192.

Page 49

3. Markham, Laura. (2013) Peaceful Parent, Happy Kids - How to stop
yelling and start connecting (Audiobook). Tantor Audio.
Retrieved from www.audible.com

Page 51

4. Morell, S. & Cowan, T. (2015). The Nourishing Traditions book of
baby & Childcare. Washington, DC: New Trends Publishing Inc., Pg.
212.

Page 53

5. Serrallach, Oscar. (2018). The Postnatal Depletion Cure. London,
Great Britain: Sphere, Pg.3-13.

Page 54

6. Pastore E, & Katzman W. (2012) Recognizing Myofascial Pelvic Pain
in the Female Patient with Chronic Pelvic Pain. Journal of Obstetric,
Gynecologic and Neonatal Nursing. 41(5), 680-691.

Chapter 4 by Naomi Haupt

Page 61

Opening quote:

Millman, Dan. Way of the Peaceful Warrior: A Book That Changes Lives. Tiburon, California: H J Kramer Inc., 2006.

Chapter 5 by Melissa Smith

Page 77

Opening quote:

Maya Angelou Quotes. BrainyQuote.com, BrainyMedia Inc, 2019. https://www.brainyquote.com/quotes/maya_angelou_120197, retrieved October 16, 2019.

Chapter 6 by Tara Butterwick

Page 89

Opening quote:

Tony Robbins. "The Danger of Expectations." https://www.tonyrobbins.com/love-relationships/the-danger-of-expectations/, retrieved October 16, 2019.

Page 91

1. S. (26, October 26). Preterm live births in Canada. Retrieved from https://www150.statcan.gc.ca/n1/pub/82-625-x/2016001/article/14675-eng.htm

Page 93

2. D. L. (2017). Diastasis Rectus Abdominis, A Clinical Guide for those who are split down the middle. Vancouver, BC: Learn

Chapter 7 by Hillary Dinning

Page 103

Opening quote:

Kornfield, Jack. Buddha's Little Instruction Book. Bantam, 1994.

Page 111

1. Glennon Doyle, "Love Is the Opposite of Control," Facebook. https://www.facebook.com/watch/?v=1612236325551352, retrieved October 16, 2019.

Page 112

2. Chicken Soup for the Soul. Chickensoup.com/book-story/40480/it-will-change-your-life, retrieved November 2019.

SECTION 2: by Sabrina Greer

Page 117

1. Brain Anatomy, Anatomy of the Human Brain. (n.d.). Retrieved from https://mayfieldclinic.com/pe-anatbrain.htm.
2. Statistics on Postpartum Depression - Postpartum Depression Resources. (n.d.). Retrieved from https://www.postpartumdepression.org/resources/statistics/.

Chapter 8 by Amanda Archibald

Page 125

Opening quote:
Brown, Brené. Daring Greatly: How the Courage to be Vulnerable Transforms the Way We Live, Love, Parent, and Lead. New York: Penguin Random House, 2012.

Chapter 9 by Tania Jane Moraes-Vaz

Page 139

Opening quote:
Murakami, Haruki. Norwegian Wood. New York: Random House, 2000.

Chapter 10 by Mona Sharma

Page 153

Opening quote:
Chopra, Deepak, and Rudolph E. Tanzi. The Healing Self: A Revolutionary New Plan to Supercharge Your Immunity and Stay Well for Life. New York: Harmony Books, 2018.

Chapter 11 by Andrea Taylor

Page 167

Opening quote:
Debbie Ford Quote. (n.d.). Retrieved from https://www.azquotes.com/quote/850874, retrieved October 16, 2019.

Page 170, 174

1. Marcoux, H. (2019, June 13). More than half of new moms aren't getting the mental health support they need. Retrieved from https://www.mother.ly/news/survey-new-moms-arent-getting-mental-health-support

Page 170

2. Birben, E., Sahiner, U. M., Sackesen, C., Erzurum, S., & Kalayci, O. (2012). Oxidative stress and antioxidant defense. The World Allergy Organization journal, 5(1), 9–19. doi:10.1097/WOX.0b013e3182439613

Page 171

3. Antidepressant Medication. (n.d.). Retrieved from https://www.camh.ca/en/health-info/mental-illness-and-addiction-index/antidepressant-medications

Page 173

4. Unfortunately. (n.d.). Diet for Depression | Foods that Help Depression. Retrieved from https://www.webmd.com/depression/guide/diet-recovery#1

Page 174

5. Kilbourne, J. (1999). Can't Buy My Love: How Advertising Changes The Way We Think and Feel. New York: Touchstone.

Page 178

6. Selhub, E. (2018, April 5). Nutritional psychiatry: Your brain on food. Retrieved from https://www.health.harvard.edu/blog/ nutritional-psychiatry-your-brain-on-food-201511168626

7. Weir, K. (2011, December). The exercise effect: Evidence is mounting for the benefits of exercise, yet psychologists don't often use exercise as part of their treatment arsenal. Here's more research on why they should. Retrieved from https://www.apa.org/monitor/2011/12/exercise

Chapter 12 by Christina Whelan Chabot

Page 185

Opening quote:

Nora Ephron Quotes. BrainyQuote.com, BrainyMedia Inc, 2019. https://www.brainyquote.com/quotes/nora_ephron_746125, retrieved October 16, 2019.

Page 188

1. Understanding the stress response: chronic activation of this survival mechanism impairs health. (2011, March). Retrieved from: www.health.harvard.edu/staying-healthy/ understanding-the-stress-response.

2. Routledge, F. S., Campbell, T. S., McFetridge-Durdle, J. S., & Bacon, S. L. (2010). Improvements in heart rate variability with exercise therapy. Canadian Journal of Cardiology, 26(6), 303-312.

3. Reed, M. J., Robertson, C. E., & Addison, P. S. (2005). Heart rate variability measurements and the prediction of ventricular arrhythmias. Quarterly Journal of Medicine, 98, 87-95.

Page 189

4. Arnsten, A. F. T. (2009). Stress signaling pathways that impair prefrontal cortex structure and function. Nature Reviews Neuroscience, 10(6), 410-422.

5. Waldstein, S. R., Kop, W. J., Schmidt, L. A., Haufler, A. J., Krantz, D.S., & Fox, N. A. (2000). Frontal electrocortical and cardiovascular reactivity during happiness and anger. Biological Psychology, 55, 3–23.

6. Schmidt, L. A., Fox, N. A., Schulkin, J., & Gold, P. W. (1999). Behavioral and psychophysiological correlates of self-presentation in temperamentally shy children. Developmental Psychobiology, 35, 119–135.

Page 190

7. Aubert A. E., Seps, B., & Beckers, F. (2003). Heart rate variability in athletes. Sports Medicine 33(12), 889-919.

Page 190

8. Sheffield D, Krittayaphong R, Cascio WE, Light KC, Golden RN, Ginkel JB, Glekas G, Koch GG, Sheps DS. Heart rate variability at rest and during mental stress in patients with coronary artery disease: differences in patients with high and low depression scores. Int J Behav Med 1998; 5: 31–47.

9. Mammen, G. & Faulkner, G. (2013). Physical activity and the prevention of depression: a systematic review of prospective studies. American Journal of Preventative Medicine, 45(5), 649-657.

10. Dunn, A. L., Trivedi, M. H., Kampert, J. B., Clark, C. G. & Chambliss, H. O. (2005). Exercise treatment for depression: Efficacy and dose response. American Journal of Preventative Medicine, 28(1), 1-8.

Page 191

11. Cumming J., Williams S. E. (2014). Imagery. In: Encyclopedia of sport and exercise psychology. Ed: Eklund R.C., Tenenbuam G., editors. Los Angeles: Sage; 369-373.

12. Slimani, M., Chamari, K., Boudhiba, D., & Cheour, F. (2016). Mediator and moderator variables of imagery use-motor learning and sport performance relationships: a narrative review. Sport Sciences for Health, 12, 1-9.

Page 191

13. Franklin, E. (2018, September 5). About Dynamic Neurocognitive Imagery (DNI)TM. Retrieved from: www.franklinmethod.com

14. 20 Franklin, E. (2018, September 5). About the Franklin Method. Retrieved from: www.franklinmethod.com

Page 192

15. Li, C., Chang, Q., Zhang, J., Chai, W. (2018). Effects of slow breathing rate on heart rate variability and arterial baroreflex sensitivity in essential hypertension. Medicine, 97(18).

16. Ma, X., Yue, Z-Q, Gong, Z-Q, Zhang, H., Duan, N-Y, Shi, Y-T, Wei, G-X & Li, Y-F. (2017). The effect of diaphragmatic breathing on attention, negative affect and stress in healthy adults. Frontiers in Psychology, 8, 874.

17. Brown, R. P. & Gerbarg, P. L. (2005). Sudarshan Kriya Yogic breathing in the treatment of stress, anxiety, and depression. Part II--clinical applications and guidelines. Journal of Alternative and Complementary Medicine, 11(4), 711-7.

18. Anju, D., Chopra, A., Jain, R., Yadav, D., Vedamurthachar. (2015). Effectiveness of yogic breathing intervention on quality of life of opioid dependent users. International Journal of Yoga, 8(2), 144-7.1

19. Russo, M. A., Santarelli, D. M., & O'Rourke, D. (2017). The physiological effects of slow breathing in the healthy human. Breathe, 13(4), 298-309.

20. Take a deep breath (2009, May). Retrieved from: www.health. harvard.edu/staying-healthy/take-a-deep-breath

21. Gerritsen, R.J.S. and Band, G.P.H. (2018). Breath of Life: The Respiratory Vagal Stimulation Model of Contemplative Activity. Frontiers in Human Neuroscience, 12: 397.

Page 189

23. Belknap, Catherine, and Natalie Telfer. Cat and Nat's Mom Truths: Embarrassing Stories and Brutally Honest Advice on the Extremely Real Struggle of Motherhood. New York: Harmony Books, 2019.

Chapter 13 by Jodi Decle

Page 199

Opening quote:
Lisa Nichols (@2Motivate), "Your job is to fill your own cup, so it overflows. Then you can serve others, joyfully, from your own saucer," Twitter, June 18, 2019, 11:14 p.m.

SECTION 3: by Sabrina Greer

Page 213

1. Weinberg, J. (2019, August 16). Mind-Body Connection: Understanding the Psycho-Emotional Roots of Disease. Retrieved from https://chopra.com/articles/mind-body-connection-understanding-the-psycho-emotional-roots-of-disease.

Chapter 14 by Danielle Williams

Page 221

Opening quote:
Glennon Doyle, https://momastery.com/blog/, retrieved October 17, 2019.

Page 226

1. McKee, T. "The Geography of Sorrow, Francis Weller on Navigating Losses." The Sun Magazine, Oct 2015, https://www.thesunmagazine.org/issues/478/the-geography-of-sorrow. 11July 2018.

Page 228

2. Zebian, Najwa. The Nectar of Pain. Kansas City, Missouri: Andrews McMeel, 2018.

Page 229

3. "Everything is a Miracle," Albert Einstein. http://www.awakin.org/read/view.php?tid=255, retrieved October 17, 2019.

Chapter 15 by Justine Dowd

Page 235

Opening quote:
Germer, Christopher K. The Mindful Path to Self-Compassion:
Freeing Yourself from Destructive Thoughts and Emotions. New York,
Guilford, 2009.

Page 237

1. Neff, K. (2003) Self-compassion: An alternative conceptualization
of a healthy attitude toward oneself, Self and Identity, 2(2), 85-101.
DOI: 10.1080/15298860309032

Page 238

2. Harter, S. (1998). The development of self-representations. In W.
Damon & N. Eisenberg (Ed.), Handbook of child psychology: Social,
emotional, and personality development (pp. 553-617). Hoboken,
NJ, US: John Wiley & Sons Inc.

Page 239

3. Swann, W. B. (1996). Self-traps: The elusive quest for higher self-
esteem. New York: Freeman.

Page 243

4. Covington, S. N., & Burns, L. H. (Eds.). (2006). Infertility
counseling: A comprehensive handbook for clinicians. Cambridge
University Press.

Page 244

5. Raque-Bogdan, T. L., & Hoffman, M. A. (2015). The relationship
among infertility, self-compassion, and well-being for women with
primary or secondary infertility. Psychology of Women Quarterly,
39(4), 484-496.

Chapter 16 by Maria Blackley

Page 253

Opening quote:

KeepInspiring.Me: Inspiration Served with a heavy dose of reality, https://www.keepinspiring.me/uplifting-quotes-for-difficult-times, retrieved October 17, 2019.

Page 255

1. What is an ectopic pregnancy? https://www.mayoclinic.org/diseases-conditions/ectopic-pregnancy/symptoms-causes/syc-20372088

Chapter 17 by Shayroz Khosla

Page 269

Opening quote:

Anthony, Mark. The Beautiful Truth. Self-published, CreateSpace, 2016.

Chapter 18 by Leisha Laird

Page 283

Opening quote:

Maya Angelou Quotes. BrainyQuote.com, BrainyMedia Inc, 2019. https://www.brainyquote.com/quotes/maya_angelou_392897, accessed October 16, 2019.

Page 285

1. "Boundaries," Brené Brown. The Work of the People: Films for Discovery & Transformation, https://www.theworkofthepeople.com/boundaries, retrieved October 11, 2019.

YGT MAMA
MEDIA CO.

HELPING MAMAS BIRTH THEIR BRAIN BABIES

At YGTMama Media Co., we help mamas bring their visions to life. Through a collaborative and supportive community, we truly value the idea that it takes a village as we bring your Brain Baby into this world. We are a unique and boutique publisher and professional branding company that caters to all stages of business around your book and personal brand as an author. We work with seasoned and emerging authors on solo and collaborative projects.

Our mamas have a safe space to grow and diversify themselves within the genres of nonfiction, personal development, spiritual enlightenment, health and wellness, love and relationships, motherhood and business as well as children's books, journals, and personal and professional growth tools. We help motivated mamas realize dreams and ideas by breathing life into their powerful passions. We believe in women's empowerment, community over competition, and equal opportunity. You are so much more than "just a mom." **You've got this, Mama!**

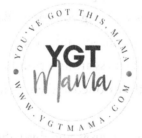

JOIN OR CONNECT WITH THE MAMA TRIBE

YGTMAMA.COM | YGTMAMAMEDIA.CO

YGTMAMA | @YGTMAMA.MEDIA.CO

YGTMAMA | @YGTMAMA.MEDIA.CO